# Pulp Med

## Why Doctors Will Give You
## Only Half-Truths

# Pulp Med

## Why Doctors Will Give You Only Half-Truths

Petros Arguriou

and

Beldeu Singh

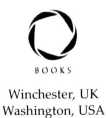

BOOKS

Winchester, UK
Washington, USA

First published by O-Books, 2011
O-Books is an imprint of John Hunt Publishing Ltd., Laurel House, Station Approach,
Alresford, Hants, SO24 9JH, UK
office1@o-books.net
www.o-books.com

For distributor details and how to order please visit the 'Ordering' section on our website.

Text copyright: Petros Arguriou and Beldeu Singh 2010

ISBN: 978 1 84694 699 8

A CIP catalogue record for this book is available from the British Library.

Design: Stuart Davies


Printed in the UK by CPI Antony Rowe
Printed in the USA by Offset Paperback Mfrs, Inc

We operate a distinctive and ethical publishing philosophy in all
areas of our business, from our global network of authors to
production and worldwide distribution.

# CONTENTS

Foreword    xi

Prologue    1

Introduction    5

Chapter 1: Magic bullets and wonder drugs    12

Chapter 2: Cancer    37

Chapter 3: Of self and others    62

Chapter 4: Towards a global health dictatorship    106

Chapter 5: Psychodictatorship    139

Chapter 6: On the legality of drugs    185

Chapter 7: Towards a new public health model    201

References    227

Bibliography    245

Authors contribution map:

Peter Arguriou: pgs xi-xii, 1-4, 12-25, 27-51, 62-74, 139-188, 215-226

Beldeu Singh: pgs 25-27, 51-61, 97-138, 189-200, 208-215

G. Vithoulkas: pgs 5-11

J. Roberts: 75-97

Mae-Wan Ho: 201-208

# About the authors

**Peter Arguriou** is an author born in the sunny city of Thessaloniki, Greece, in the summer of 1973.

He studied medicine in the University of Athens Medical School and classical homeopathy in the Aegean University.

He is a member of the Hellenic MENSA.

For a brief period of time he regrettably worked for the Greek pharmaceutical industry.

For several years now has been writing for the Greek Press about the real story behind public health policies and news.

He also writes periodically for *Nexus Magazine*.

His upcoming book "Novel epidemics and the medical apocalypse" is expected to be released in late 2012

You can contact Peter through his personal blog (http://hellasashell.wordpress.com)

**Beldeu Singh** is a physical anthropologist with a wide scope of expertise covering training and development, marketing to law and from management to antioxidants and nanobiotechnology in medicine with an active interest in human biochemistry and drugless therapies. He is also author of a novel and a book on insurance law. He maintains an academic interest in politics.

# Contributing Authors

**George Vithoulkas** was born in Athens in July 25, 1932. He is Professor of Homeopathic Medicine, Honorary Professor of the Moscow Medical Academy (Academy of Medical Sciences) , Professor in the Kiev Medical Academy and Collaborating Professor in Basque Medical University (2001-2004).

In 1996, he was honored with the Right Livelihood Award (also known as Alternative Nobel Prize, "...for his outstanding contribution to the revival of homeopathic knowledge and the training of homeopaths to the highest standards." The United Nations (Development Forum) considers this award "Among the world's most prestigious awards", while TIME Magazine called Jakob von Uexkull, the award's inspirator, as one of the 37 "heroes" of 2005. In 2000, George Vithoulkas was honored with the Gold Medal of the Hungarian Republic from the country's president, Arpad Goncz, for his work in the homeopathic medicine.

In 1995, he established International Academy of Classical Homeopathy in Alonissos, in which he is the director. In this academy, George Vithoulkas gives the gist of 40 years of his experience and his recent ideas of levels of health. In his teachings, he gives details that will help the doctor to determine the state of health of each individual patient and also the possibility to be estimated whether a case is curable with homeopathy, and the amount of time and remedies that will be needed to accomplish a cure.

**Dr. Mae-Wan Ho** was born in Hong Kong on November 12, 1941. Ho received a Ph.D. in Biochemistry in 1967 from Hong Kong University, was Postdoctoral Fellow in Biochemical Genetics, University of California San Diego from 1968 to 1972, Senior Research Fellow in Queen Elizabeth College, Lecturer in Genetics (from 1976) and Reader in Biology (from 1985) in the Open University, and a Visiting Professor of Biophysics in Catania University, Sicily (from 2000). Dr. Mae-Wan Ho is best known for pioneering work on the physics of organisms and sustainable systems; she is also a critic of genetic engineering biotechnology and neo-Darwinism. She is Director and co-founder of the Institute of Science in Society (www.i-sis.org.uk), and Editor-in-Chief and Art Director of its trend-setting quarterly magazine *Science in Society.*

She has more than 170 scientific publications and over 500 popular articles. Her books include Beyond Neo-Darwinism: An

Introduction to the New Evolutionary Paradigm (1984); Evolutionary Processes and Metaphors (1988); The Rainbow and the Worm, the Physics of Organisms (1993, $2^{nd}$ ed.1998, reprinted 1999, 2001, 2003, 2005; 2006, $3^{rd}$ ed, 2008); Bioelectrodynamics and Biocommunication (1994), Bioenergetics (1995); Genetic Engineering Dream or Nightmare? (1998, 1999, reprint with extended introduction, 2007); Living with the Fluid Genome (2003); The Case for a GM-Free Sustainable World (2003, 2004); Unravelling AIDS (2005); Which Energy? (2006), Food Futures Now (2008)

**Janine Roberts** is an investigative journalist, author and filmmaker. Her work as an investigative journalist has appeared in the Melbourne Age, Sydney Morning Herald, The Independent, Independent on Sunday, Financial Times and many other papers and periodicals. She has also produced investigative films shown on the BBC, Channel Four, Frontline (WGBH) in the USA, ABC's Four Corners in Australia and on a project with Panorama, BBC. She has also initiated and researched a World in Action for Grenada TV and made an independent film that won a Best Documentary Nomination.

She has authored/edited three books on the plight of Australian Aborigines, with her work being used by John Pilger. Her work on blood diamonds in "Glitter and Greed" and "The Diamond Empire" led to her being invited to testify at a US Congressional Hearing.

Her latest investigative work on vaccines and infectious diseases is "Fear of the Invisible". It has been widely cited internationally, shows further possible links of vaccines to autism, citing as evidence previously undisclosed transcripts of top governmental scientists' meetings – and has led to a letter from 37 scientists and doctors in December 2008 to the Science journal calling for the withdrawal of key HIV research papers on the grounds of fraud.

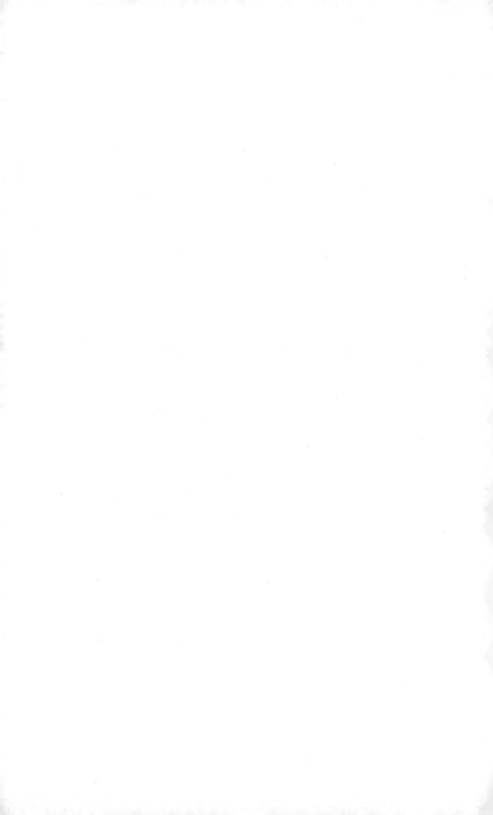

# Foreword

The book you are holding is an outcome of decades of dedicated research, research done by dozens of individuals, a lot of times challenged or challenging mainstream medicine. It is a collective work that couldn't have been materialized without the contribution and the magnanimity of alternative medical pioneers. Now, being alternative does not necessarily mean being right, the claim of omniscience is far beyond the scopes of this book, or its contributors. It is only natural that the authors do not necessarily agree with each other on everything and that every author is exclusively responsible for the opinions he expresses. The scope of this book is not to present the reader with a consensus but to present him with a wide spectrum of opinions, health approaches and health tips. It is not about instructing, or mandating, or about replacing the current medical dictatorship with an alternative one. It is about informing the reader about sources that he would hardly have any access to. It is about presenting a confused and dissatisfied "medical consumer" with options, empowering him to make his own choices over health and disease.

Some contributors and some articles may appear controversial. So be it. It is high time that all interested parties drop the facade of omniscience and the garment of self-interest, and engage in a fruitful public health dialogue. The time is ripe not only for a general, public health policy reform but for a deep medical science and funds reform also. And this can only be achieved through social health movements. After decades of just and justified forms of political activism, it is high time that activism expands in the public health domain.

I would like to thank first of all my wonderful co-writer, Beldeu Singh. Working with him has been a blessing. I would also like to thank the contributing authors for the trust and care they vested in this book. I can only hope that you, the readers, find the effort and time invested in this book worth your while.

P.A

# Prologue

We live in an era of crisis. That much is obvious. What has eluded us is that the crisis is not merely a financial one and not exclusively an environmental one. It is also a deep cultural crisis with humanity in its totality being unable to envision a future or to shape viable and motivating ideas and ideals.

In this age, the only aspect of human endeavor that has not been deeply wounded by doubt, which has escaped criticism, is science. The main reason for this exemption is that science is presented as an autonomous domain governed by its own rules and principles, namely by SCIENTIFIC TRUTH. But in fact, nothing could be further from the truth.

Science is also a social product and it is deeply affected by the zeitgeist, the preeminent mentality of an epoch, by stereotypes, practices and notions that permeate an era.

If this applies to science in general, its implications for medicine expand even further. Because medicine is not even an exact science like physics or chemistry. There is no great theory of life or health. Some somatic mechanisms have been explained, others have not.

Medicine is even further burdened by trends and fashions in science.

The ultra specialization and the acute clustering of knowledge and research that was necessary to accelerate progress became a problem in its own right. We increased the velocity, the altitude and the capacity of modern research but we forgot how to perform. That led to an oxymoron. The more information we got from the ultra specialized science, the less able we were to combine it and transform it into a meaningful scientific corpus. It is easy to dissect a living organism into tiny bits to see how it works, but it is almost impossible to reassemble it and reanimate it. That is what happened to us. That is why we are failing in pressing medical issues. We were so taken by the tree, so focused on it, that we lost view of the forest. We failed to see the *Big Picture*.

Without a meaningful overview of medical research and industry, major oversights and faults were bound to happen.

And off course they did happen.

We still don't know what cancer exactly is. We know what cancer cells are and sometimes we know how they behave, but we don't know what cancer actually is.

We don't know what causes autoimmune diseases. We kind of know how they occur but we don't know exactly why and when they occur and how to treat them.

We don't know exactly how HIV and other viruses create pathology; we don't know the exact mechanisms. Come to think of it we don't know what a virus actually is, what its exact role in the microenvironment is, we don't know its phylogenesis and origins.

We know about proteins, genes, specific markers and other biomolecules in mind-blowing details, but we are unable to give satisfying answers to pressing medical questions. Indeed, it is the tree we are seeing and not the forest. And that wouldn't be happening if there was a great underlying medical theory, if there was a consistent medical philosophy able to provide us with the framework for the unbelievable sum of information we have acquired.

We still don't know what life exactly is, we don't know what death exactly is. We can't for example define the exact moment when the transition from inanimate matter to animate occurs and vice versa. We can't tell the exact point in time when a fertilized cell becomes a living entity, that is, when life begins; we can't tell the exact point in time when a living entity ceases to be alive, that is when life ends. And these issues, life and death issues, contrary to what is commonly believed, are not moral, they should not be defined by moral considerations. They are predominantly scientific ones. Modern medicine fails to answer fundamental questions about life, death, health and disease, yet it claims to own an unparalleled know-how regarding health and disease, to claim to exert control over them when it can hardly define or understand them.

Overspecialization combined with a complete absence of an underlying medical philosophy is only one side of the coin. When it is flipped over, the other great inadequacy of medicine instantly appears: medicine suffers also from over generalization and over simplification. Modern medicine has created a "communist" concept and model of public health. It has invented the "median" man or patient and directed all of its energies towards that imaginary median man. Yes, all men are equal and the human biochemistry is generally the same but all humans are definitely not identical in body composition, blood antioxidant levels and in their genetic make-up. Granted, organisms belonging to the same species have lots in common but they are not in any conceivable way identical. This "communist" medicine, this populist medicine, this Pulp Medicine knows of no borders. It has dominated medical thought, research and practice all over the world. When it comes to health and sickness, individuality is leveled. It is all about mass sales and huge markets composed of billions of those "median" people. It is fueled by a raw material that comes at no cost and in plentitude called sickness and it thrives at our expense. It is the business of Pulp Med exactly because it uses people as pulp, a homogenous mass waiting to be treated even if they cannot be helped and shaped into wellness.

Pulp Med is not only treating people bad, it is also treating science bad. Besides resorting to overspecialization and overgeneralization, Pulp Med is also full of medical anomalies. Deviations from what we would have normally anticipated pop up where they are least expected, constantly denying Pulp Med credibility and validity. We choose to turn a blind eye on them.

We choose to systematically ignore the "miraculous" spontaneous healing even in terminal patients. We ascribe to it the vague term self-healing and hurriedly close the discussion. We give a name to the astonishing phenomenon of people responding to inactive "dummy" pills; we call it placebo and we sweep it under the carpet.

But before we enter the structural anomalies of medicine we have first to explore its fundamental scientific deficiency: the lack of an underlying medical philosophy. It is exactly this Pulp Med birth defect that has resulted to an inability to shape a vital and absolutely necessary definition, a complete and thorough definition of Health. In our rush and willingness to combat illness we completely disregarded wellness.

# Definition and Measure of Health

The first task of a science that claims its primary aim is to restore health should be to define what "health" is, what the target or goal of treatment is, and in what direction the patient should be guided during his treatment.

One should also define the parameters for measuring health. This should be defined so that anybody can easily ascertain whether an individual under treatment is progressing toward health or is actually regressing toward a deeper state of imbalance.

I doubt whether any medical graduate could provide these definitions; I also doubt that medical students are taught to recognize an ideal state of health or to identify the parameters that measure it.

When the pain is gone, when the inflammation has subsided, when a bothersome symptom has disappeared, when the pathology is no longer evident, the patient usually is pronounced cured. Yet there may be long-term disturbances caused by the treatment, especially in deeper or more subtle parts of the human organism such as the immune or hormonal systems or, even worse, in the mental or emotional planes, that are not taken into consideration. A treatment therefore should have a beneficial effect *simultaneously* on all these levels in order to claim that it is the right kind of treatment.

Treating the whole person, which is now accepted on a rhetorical level by everyone, should be more than a theoretical dictum; it should be an applied reality.

*The Definition of Health for the Physical Body*
Disease, whether expressed through pain, discomfort or weakness, always tends to restrict the individual. Its opposite, health, gives a sense of freedom. This is the reason why in the definition that follows I have used the word "freedom" as a key word.

I also give a separate definition of health for each of the three planes since I know that an individual can be sick on one level while on another level he may appear completely healthy. For example, a schizophrenic that is deeply disturbed in his mental-emotional plane appears to be extremely healthy in his physical body. It is a well-established fact that severely mentally ill patients almost never get sick with physical ailments, even under the most adverse conditions, while others that suffer from physical ailments can be very healthy in their emotional and mental spheres.

As we have already stated, every pain, discomfort, uneasiness, distress or weakness of the physical body results in a limitation of freedom and a feeling of bondage to the pain or discomfort. The individual necessarily directs all his attention to the pain, to the exclusion of everything else, and of course loses his general sense of well-being. It is for this reason that health on the physical plane can be defined as follows: health is freedom from pain in the physical body, having attained a state of well-being.

*The Definition of Health on the Emotional Plane*
On the emotional plane, that which enslaves the individual and absorbs all his attention is excessive passion – passion in the broadest sense and not with only a sensual connotation.

Excessive, inordinate passion for anything shows a degree of imbalance within the emotional plane. For instance, when an overwhelming erotic passion for another person reaches a point where murdering this person is contemplated because of jealousy, we definitely have a disease state rather than a love state. Passion for a cause, even a lofty one that brings the individual to the point where he contemplates destructive actions against others, is definitely a diseased state rather than justified ideal-ism. A healthy state of the emotions never goes so far as to bring about destruction, but rather tries to follow the "golden mean" of the ancient Greeks.

Fanatical and dogmatic attitudes that divorce themselves from logic and understanding show a degree of unhealthy emotional involvement that usually results in some type of catastrophe, either for the individual or for others. Passionately loving somebody may mean that the degree of attachment is so great that if the love is not reciprocated the individual may commit some kind of crime (homicide or suicide).

We too often mistake our emotional needs and insecurities for real love and affection. The latter two presuppose giving without reservation. It is emotional attachment that constantly makes demands of others under the pretence of giving. Certainly the opposite of passion – apathy – is no more desirable. Apathy is an extremely unhealthy emotional state, very much akin to the idea of death. What is desirable is a state of serenity and calm that is dynamic and creative, not passive, indifferent or destructive – a state where love and positive emotions prevail, as opposed to hatred and other negative emotions.

In order to justify their origin and destiny, human beings have to transcend their animal nature, and have to make **conscious efforts to evolve**, not so much in their physical body as in their mental and emotional spheres.

I believe that it is clear now that (*obsessive*) passion comes from weakness rather than strength on the emotional plane. Thus the definition for this plane should be: health on the emotional plane is freedom from (obsessive) passion, having as a result a dynamic state of serenity and calm.

*The Definition of Health on the Mental-Spiritual Plane*
To give a concise definition of health on the mental-spiritual plane is a rather difficult task because one must identify the most important mental-spiritual qualities, which if disturbed may seriously injure the mental equilibrium.

After much deliberation I have come to the conclusion that peace of mind can be drastically affected by egotism, selfishness and acquisitiveness. The more egotistical and selfish an individual is, the greater his potential for mental derangement.

It is a known fact that a person who is very egotistical can be quite upset when his authority, knowledge or attainments are challenged. A humble man with the same attainments will hardly react to the unjust criticism of others, and will actually see the positive side of the criticism and correct his course of action accordingly. The same "shocks" that can set off an egotist and destroy him can leave a humble man almost unaffected.

An egotistical industrialist who fails in his business and loses his factory cares more about the opinion that others now have of him than the fate of the families, including his own, that will have no means to support themselves. It is his ego that has been hurt. Even if he has plenty to live on without the factory, he will feel miserable after the failure and is bound to develop a host of symptoms because of his "false" and selfish grief.

In a similar way, acquisitiveness could become the core of mental disturbance. Can you imagine how an avaricious man might react to the loss of his physical wealth and the deep symptomatology that could result?

Hardly anyone today is totally free from the feelings of egotism, selfishness and acquisitiveness.

It is also a fact that the person engrossed in his own ego can neither see objectively nor perceive the truth. He thinks he always knows everything and knows it better than anyone else. Humanity has suffered great disasters because of such attitudes. Looking back in history we frequently recognize this quality and label it insanity.

We speak about the insanity of Hitler, Idi Amin Dada, even of the captain in charge of the Titanic whose arrogance cost the lives of hundreds. In our own way, every one of us is dealing with similar issues on a smaller scale. This "disease" called egotism and selfishness seems to be universal. That is why we are so likely to admire and worship the saints; we believe that they actually managed to subdue their egotism and sacrifice their own lives for the sake of others. We worship them as "superior" human beings because their accomplishment seems beyond our comprehension. Although rare, this "saint-like" attitude is the healthiest to possess; in such a state true peace of mind and happiness is achieved.

It is peculiar, though, that this state of health can only be achieved through conscious efforts of the individual, while the state of health of the physical body is a birthright.

There is a natural legacy and an inherent urge for human beings to evolve into people of "Love and Wisdom". Only with a New Model for Health and Disease will there be hope for the human race. Not until we start seeing the issue in all of its dimensions will there be hope for a better state of health.

This imbalance we feel on the mental-spiritual plane is perhaps the most challenging and complicated issue we have to face. Nobody is exempt from this imbalance, though there are different degrees. The greater an individual's egotism and selfishness, the greater are his possibilities for a mental breakdown.

We can therefore define mental health as: freedom from selfishness in the mental sphere, having as a result total unification with Truth.

So now we summarize the whole definition of Health: health is freedom from pain in the physical body, a state of well-being; freedom from passion on the emotional plane, resulting in a dynamic state of serenity and calm; and freedom from selfishness in the mental sphere, having as a result total unification with Truth. A truly healthy individual should therefore combine both divine qualities of Love and Wisdom.

It is obvious that such a state of health is an ideal and that nobody can possess it in its entirety; but the definition points to an ideal *Model* of health toward which therapeutic treatments should aspire. The more a patient under treatment approaches this state, the healthier he becomes; and the more he moves away from it, the less healthy he becomes.

*The Measure of Health*

It is obvious at this point that we need some parameters to measure health.

Some questions are required of us. For example: if we cure somebody of asthma and as a consequence he develops a heart condition, how do we know that this new state of health is better or worse than his previous condition? If we treat a patient with a cardiac condition and he improves, but after a certain period of time he develops a phobic state or an anxiety neurosis, can we say that the treatment benefited the patient?

We shall see that in order for a treatment to be successful it has to push the disorder's center of gravity more and more to the peripheral, the skin being the final avenue of expression, leaving the deepest parts of the human being – his mental and emotional levels – intact.

As I have said, the issue of determining an individual's exact degree of health is a complicated task requiring much research and involving a number of parameters before precise answers are possible. But as a general rule of thumb, we can say that a good parameter for measuring the health of an individual is the degree to which he is free to create. Anybody who is basically healthy will seek to create rather than destroy. By creativity, as I have stated previously, I mean all those actions that promote the interests and good of oneself and others. To the degree that one commits destructive acts toward either himself or others, the degree to which he is diseased is apparent.

*Pulp Med does not only lack essential and complete definitions of health as it is a disease-oriented discipline. It also lacks focus on real-time and pragmatic health. An agriculturist will tell you the optimum conditions for growing plants, a vet will give you advice on how to raise a healthy pet but your doctor won't tell you what to do to preserve or increase your health. And that's quite expected as he is trained to combat disease, not to boost health. Pulp Med as a whole is defined and confined by such a gargantuan deficiency. And this enormous gap has to be properly addressed by a more competent approach and philosophy. The most likely candidate to fill this fundamental absence is the field of medicine that examines health at a very fundamental level, at the cellular level, combined with other holistic disciplines that embrace a systemic approach towards the organism, regarding it as more than a sum of its parts.*

*Chapter I*

# Magic bullets and wonder drugs

*We need to find a way to measure health at every level, from social and public health, to individual and even cellular health. Yet few invest effort to achieve such a goal. One could say that since we are incapable or unwilling to introduce proper measurements of health, we should stick to what we know best: that is, measure and evaluate therapy. And the most tangible part of measuring a therapy is to test the drugs when and if they are involved in therapy.*

*We have been evaluating drug toxicity and efficacy for so long that by now we should be confident of our mastery over it. So it would be kind of surprising to hear someone proclaim drug evaluations unreliable. Shocking or not, under the current drug evaluation system we can be certain about most of the drugs only from empirical data amassed after years or even decades of safe and expedient use.*

*There are many reasons behind the drug testing elusiveness. An outstanding one is a phenomenon that has been poorly understood or totally misunderstood: placebo is incorporated and used as a criterion for drug evaluation while at the same time it induces the placebo effect, a systematic medical anomaly. In other words, we are measuring drugs and testing them against something that is definitely not a golden standard but rather a variable that can not be standardized or normalized or predicted. That means that all placebo-controlled drug evaluations are inaccurate by nature. The placebo effect tampers with drugs profiles as much as bias. No wonder drugs are being withdrawn years after their initial approval.*

*The drug approval system itself needs to be revisited and revamped. All drugs must be tested for their toxicity and for their toxic effects on mineral depletion, immune suppression, vitamin C depletion, suppression of coenzyme Q10 production, glutathione depletion and their potential to mediate genetic damage. All drugs must undergo tests that reveal their capacity to generate free radicals especially ROS in cellular systems. This information must be provided to doctors so that they are put in a better position to advise their patients rather than dish out half-truths.*

*Another important test is to study the effects of drugs on the symbiotic flora in the gut. Symbiotic bacteria produce butyric acid and other useful molecules. These symbiotic bacteria also help to keep Candida in check. Their destruction can lead to health problems. Hence, the need for probiotic medicine as a post-drug therapy in the proper restoration of health.*

*Currently, a drug company may conduct a number of clinical studies but it is required to submit only two studies. Most often and invariably, the drug companies will submit only the two most favorable studies.*

*All of these measures are vital if not critical in order to have greater drug safety and in order to reduce the number of adverse drug reactions (ADRs) that occur in the ten thousands every year worldwide. Wherever possible the therapy to reverse side effects of drugs and their adverse reactions must be stated. This will also reduce lawsuits and insurance payouts.*

## a) Why doctors will give you only half-truths about...
## The Placebo Effect:
## The Missing Link in Medical Evolution

*A neglected phenomenon*

One of the most commonly used terms in medical language is the word *placebo*. The *placebo effect* is used as a scale for evaluating the effectiveness of new drugs. But what exactly is the placebo effect and what are its consequences in the deterministic structure of Western medicine? The placebo effect has been frequently abused by health professionals to denote and stigmatize a fraud or fallacy. Alternative therapies have often been characterized as merely placebos. But the placebo effect is not a fraudulent, useless or malevolent phenomenon. It occurs independently of the intentions of charlatans or health professionals. It is a spontaneous, authentic and very factual phenomenon that refers to well-observed but uninterpreted and contingent therapies or health improvements that occur in the absence of an active chemical/pharmacological substance. Make-believe drugs – drugs that carry no active chemical substances – often act as real drugs and provoke therapeutic effects when administered to patients. In many drug trials, the manufacturers of the drug sadly discover that their product is in no way superior to the effect of a placebo. But that does not mean that a placebo equates to a null response of the human organism. On the contrary, a placebo denotes nonchemical stimuli that strongly motivate the organism towards a therapeutic path. That is, the placebo effect is dependent not on the drug effectivity but solely on therapeutic intention and expectation.

*Effects of positive and negative thinking*
The placebo effect has been often misunderstood as a solely psychological and highly subjective phenomenon. The patient, convinced of the therapy's effectiveness, ignores his symptoms or perceives them faintly without any substantial improvement of his health; that is, the patient *feels* better but is not healthier. But can the subjective psychological aspect of the placebo effect account for all of its therapeutic properties? The answer is definite: the placebo effect refers to an alternative curative mechanism that is inherent in the human entity, is motivated by therapeutic intention or belief in the therapeutic potential of a treatment, and induces biochemical responses and reactions to the stimulus of therapeutic intention or belief.

But placebos are not always beneficial: they can also have adverse effects. For example, administering a pharmacologically inactive substance to some patients can sometimes bring about unexpected health deteriorations. A review of 109 double-blind studies estimated that 19% of placebo recipients manifested the *nocebo* effect: unexpected deteriorations of health.[1] In a related experiment, researchers falsely declared to the volunteers that a weak electrical current would pass through their head; although there was no electrical current, 70% of the volunteers (who were medical students) complained of a headache after the experiment.[2]

In a group of patients suffering from carotid atherosclerosis, prognosis and progression of the disease were burdened when their psychological health was bad (i.e., they were affected by hopelessness or depression). In another group of carotid atherosclerosis patients, prognosis and progression were burdened not only by hopelessness but also by hostility.[3] In patients with coronary heart disease, hopelessness was a determinative risk factor.[4] Social isolation, work stress and hostility comprised additional risk factors.[5]

Positive or negative thinking seems to be a decisive risk factor for every treatment, perhaps even more important than medical intervention.

The nocebo effect appears to have a specific biological substrate. A group of 15 men whose wives suffered from terminal cancer participated in a small perspective study. After their wives' deaths, the men experienced severe grief that caused immunodepression. The spouses' lymphocytes for a period of time after their wives' deaths responded poorly to mitogens.

Grief had assaulted their immune system. The study proposed that grief and grief-induced immunodepression resulted in increased mortality in the specific group.[6]

*A short history of a small miracle*
The term *placebo* (meaning "I shall please") was used in mediaeval prayer in the context of the phrase *Placebo Domino* ("I shall please the Lord") and originated from a biblical translation

of the fifth century AD.[7] During the 18th century, the term was adopted by medicine and was used to imply preparations of no therapeutic value that were administered to patients as "decoy drugs". The term began to transform in 1920 (Graves),[8] and through various intermediate stages (Evans and Hoyle, 1933;[9] Gold, Kwit and Otto, 1937;[10] Jellinek, 1946[11]) was fully transformed in 1955 when it finally claimed an important portion of the therapeutic effect in general. Henry K. Beecher, in his 1955 paper "The Powerful Placebo", attributed a rough percentage of 30% of the overall therapeutic benefit to the placebo effect.[12] In certain later studies, placebo effect estimates were even higher, claiming 60% of the overall therapeutic outcome. In a recent review of 39 studies regarding the effectiveness of antidepressant drugs, psychologist Guy Sapirstein concluded that 50% of the therapeutic benefits came from the placebo effect, with a mere percentage of 27% attributed to drug intervention (fluoxetine, sertaline and paroxetine). Three years later Sapirstein, along with his fellow psychologist Irving Kirsch, processed the data from 19 double-blind studies regarding depression and reached an even higher percentage of therapeutic results attributed to the placebo effect: 75% depression therapies or ameliorations were placebo induced![13]

Hróbjartsson and Gotzsche (2001,[14] 2004[15]) doubted the effectiveness of the placebo phenomenon, attributing it solely to the subjective factors of human psychology. And indeed, there is a major aspect of the placebo effect related to psychology. In two studies where placebos were exclusively administered, the placebo effect seemed to be effected from the subject's perception of the applied therapy, i.e., two placebo pills were better than one, bigger pills were better than smaller, and injections were even better.[16] The placebo induced a reaction not only to the therapy but also to its form, suggesting that the placebo phenomenon is shaped according to the personal symbolic universe of the patient. Before the placebo response occurs, human perception has already interpreted the applied therapy and has prepared a certain response to it. It would appear that not only chemical but also non-chemical stimuli participate in the motivation of the human organism towards therapy. But is the placebo reaction solely a psychological phenomenon or does it have additional tangible somatic effects? One of the more dramatic events regarding placebo therapy was reported in 1957 when a new wonder drug, Krebiozen, held promise as the final solution to the cancer problem. A patient with metastatic tumors and with fluid collection in his lungs, that demanded the daily intake of oxygen and the use of an oxygen mask, heard of Krebiozen. His doctor was participating in Krebiozen research and the patient begged him to be given the revolutionary drug. Bent by the patient's hopelessness, the doctor did so and witnessed a miraculous recovery of the patient. His tumors melted and he returned to an almost normal lifestyle.

The recovery didn't last long. The patient read articles reporting on Krebiozen *not* delivering what it promised in cancer therapy. After hearing the bad news the patient had a relapse; his tumors were back. His doctor, deeply affected by the aggravation, resorted to a desperate trick. He told his patient that he had in his possession a new, improved version of Krebiozen. It was simply distilled water. The patient fully recovered after the placebo treatment and remained functional for two months. The final verdict on Krebiozen, published in the press, proved the drug to be totally ineffective. That was the *coup de grâce* for the patient, who died a few days later.[17] Although the Krebiozen case was dramatic, there is no single case or personal testimony that can denote or prove a therapy to be effective. Statistical studies, not personal testimonies, can verify a proposed therapy's effectiveness, and well planned studies are able to concur that the placebo phenomenon has somatic properties. One such study was was performed in 1997. The two study groups consisted of patients with benign prostatic hypertrophy.

One group took actual medication while the control group received placebo treatment. The placebo recipients reported relief from their symptoms and even amelioration of their urinary function.[18] A placebo has also been reported to act as a bronchodilator in asthmatic patients, or to have the exact opposite action—respiratory depression—depending on the description of the pharmacological effect the researchers gave to the patients and therefore the effect the patients anticipated.[19] A placebo proved highly efficient against food allergies and, subsequently, impressively effective in the sinking of biotechnologies on the stock market. How could that be? Peptide Therapeutics Group, a biotech company, was preparing to launch onto the market a novel vaccine for food allergies. The initial reports were encouraging. When the experimental vaccine reached the clinical trials stage, the company's spokesperson boasted that the vaccine proved effective in 75% of the cases—a percentage that usually suffices to prove a drug's effectiveness. But the good news didn't last long. The control group, given a placebo, did almost as well: seven out of 10 patients reported getting rid of their food allergies. The stock value of the company plunged by 33%. The placebo effect on food allergies created a nocebo effect on the stock market![20] In another case, a genetically designed heart drug that raised high hopes for Genentech was clobbered by a placebo.[21] As aptly put by science historian Anne Harrington, placebos are "ghosts that haunt our house of biomedical objectivity and expose the paradoxes and fissures in our own self-created definitions of the real and active factors in treatment."[22] The placebo's pharmacomimetic behavior can even imitate a drug's side effects. In a 1997 study of patients with benign prostate hypertrophy, some patients on a placebo complained of various side effects ranging from impotence and reduced sexual activity to nausea, diarrhea and constipation. Another study reported more placebo side effects as including headaches, vomiting, nausea and a variety of other symptoms.[23]

*The placebo effect in surgery*

But how deep can the placebo effect trespass into the well-defined area of medicine? Surely it can't joust with medicine's strike force; it cannot challenge surgery. Or can it? In 1939, an Italian surgeon named Davide Fieschi invented a new technique for treating angina pectoris (chest pain due to ischemia or lack of blood/oxygen getting to the heart muscle, usually due to obstruction of the coronary arteries).[24] Reasoning that increased blood flow to the heart would reduce his patients' pain, he performed tiny incisions in their chests and tied knots on the two internal mammary arteries. Three quarters of the patients showed improvement; one quarter of them was cured. The surgical intervention became standard procedure for the treatment of angina for the next 20 years. But in 1959, a young cardiologist, Leonard Cobb, put the Fieschi procedure to the test. He operated on 17 patients: on eight of them he followed the standard procedure; on the other nine he performed only the tiny incisions, letting the patients believe that they'd had the real thing. The result was a real upset: those who'd had the sham surgery did as well as those who'd had the Fieschi technique.[25] That was the end of the Fieschi technique and the beginning of the documented surgical placebo effect.

In 1994, surgeon J. Bruce Moseley experimented with the surgical placebo. He split a small group of patients suffering from osteoarthritis of the knee into two groups. Both groups were told that they would undergo arthroscopic surgery, but only the first group got the real thing. The other group was left virtually untreated, with the doctor performing only tiny incisions to make the arthroscopic scenario credible. Similar results were reported in both groups.[26] Moseley, stunned by the outcome, decided to perform the trial with a larger statistical sample in order to reach safer conclusions. The results were replicated: arthroscopic surgery was equal therapeutically to the placebo effect.[27] The placebo had found its way into surgical rooms. Perhaps the most impressive aspect of surgical placebo arose in a groundbreaking 2004 study. In the innovative field of stem-cell research, a new approach was taken with Parkinson's disease. Human embryonic dopamine neurons were implanted through tiny holes in the patients' brains. Once again, the results were encouraging. And once again, the procedure failed to do better than a placebo. In this case, the placebo involved tiny holes incised in the skull without implantation of stem cells. As the researchers confessed, "The placebo effect was very strong in this study."[28] But how can it be that the therapeutic expectancy alone can produce results that can sometimes compete with the benefits of actual surgery? It appears that the mind is exerting control over somatic processes, including diseases. The biochemical traces of this influence are only beginning to be outlined. Modern research indicates a biological, tangible substrate to the placebo effect.

*Somatic pathways*

In the mid-1990s, researcher Fabrizio Benedetti conducted a novel experiment whereby he deliberately induced ischemic pain and to sooth it with morphine administration. When morphine was replaced by a saline solution, the placebo presented analgesic properties. However, when naloxone (an opiate antagonist) was added to the saline solution, the analgesic properties of the water were blocked. Benedetti reached the conclusion that the placebo's analgesic properties were a result of specific biochemical paths. Naloxone blocked not only morphine but also endogenous opioids—the physical pain relievers.[29] The endogenous opioids, endorphins, were discovered in 1974 and act as pain antagonists. Benedetti's suggestion of a placebo-induced release of endorphins was supported by findings produced by MRI and PET scans.[30] Placebo-induced endorphin release also affects heart rate and respiratory activity.[31] As researcher Jon-Kar Zubieta described, "...this [finding] deals another serious blow to the idea that the placebo effect is a purely psychological, not physical, phenomenon."[32] Further findings support the notion that the placebo effect presents a biochemical substrate in depression and Parkinson's disease. Analyzing the results of PET scans, researchers estimated the glucose metabolism in the brains of patients with depression. Glucose metabolism under placebo presented differentiations that were similar to those caused by antidepressants such as fluoxetine.[33] In patients suffering from Parkinson's disease, a placebo injection promoted dopamine secretion in a similar way to that caused by amphetamine administration.[34] Benedetti demonstrated that the placebo effect provoked decreased activity in single neurons of the subthalamic nucleus in patients with Parkinson's disease.[35] From numerous research findings, it is logical and rather safe to conclude that there is a biochemical substrate to the placebo effect. But what is more intriguing to it is its relation to perception. It would appear that perception and the codes and symbols that the animate computer, the brain, utilizes in order to process internal and external information strongly determine the potency and form of placebo response. In a recent study, patients were purposely misinformed that they had been infected by hazardous bacilli and they subsequently underwent treatment. However, there were no bacilli and the treatment administered was a placebo. Guess what? Some of the study subjects developed infection-like conditions that were not treatable by the placebo medication.[36] The mind interpreted the fictional bacilli as hazardous and instructed the body to respond to them as if they were real.

Despite the placebo's potency and its importance for a new perception of health where body and mind heavily interact, large numbers of scientists continue to regard the placebo as an insignificant systematic error, a troublesome nought. According to cancer researcher Gershom Zajicek: "There is nothing in the pharmacokinetic theory which accounts for the placebo effect. In order to keep the theory consistent, the placebo effect is regarded as random error or noise which can be ignored."[37]

One of the most perceptive placebo researchers was Stewart Wolf, "the father of psychosomatic medicine", who as early as 1949 had given it a thorough description. Wolf not only defended the placebo as a non-fictional and very "real" phenomenon but also described the placebo's pharmacomimetic behavior. He was perhaps the first researcher to correlate the placebo effect not only with psychology and predisposition but also with perception. More than half a century ago, he stated that "The mechanisms of the body are capable of reacting not only to direct physical and chemical stimulation but also to symbolic stimuli, words and events which have somehow acquired special meaning for the individual."[38] In this context, a pill is not merely an active substance but also a therapeutic symbol and thus the organism is able to respond not only to its chemical content but also to its symbolic content. Likewise a bacillus, beyond its physical properties, acquires symbolic properties that can provoke an organism's reaction even in the absence of the bacillus. The presence and extent of the nocebo effect should also be studied in regard to drug resistance. Perhaps drug resistance is a multifactorial phenomenon involving not only microbial evolutionary aptness but also human psyche mechanics. Placebo and nocebo phenomena might prove fundamental not only on the personal level but also in the public health arena. They might even provide the foundation stone for a new model of health, a new medicine that was envisioned by Wolf in the 1950s: "...in the future, drugs will be assessed not only with reference to their pharmacologic action but also to the other forces at play and to the circumstances surrounding their administration."[39]

Five centuries ago, Swiss alchemist and physician Paracelsus (1493–1541) wrote: "You must know that the will is a powerful adjuvant of medicine." It seems that our scientific arrogance has blinded us to the teachings of the past.

## b) Why doctors will give you only half-truths about...
## The Magic Pill Effect

Theoretically, it works like a charm: people have high hopes regarding health, the drug companies eagerly and readily capitalize on people's hopes and turn them into high expectations which people in turn embrace all too willingly. This is the wonder-drug bazaar, the medical circus, a place where anything can happen, from treating acme to achieving longevity. All it takes is faith and some money. Therapy is just a clinical trial phase away.

Not quite so. In real life, most drugs and therapeutic approaches don't live up to their expectations.

And there is a good reason why this is happening. It is because of the mind-blowing and inherent complexity of every single living creature and of the diversity of every single biological entity.

Health and most of the time sickness is the combined result of innumerable factors and conditions located inside and outside the organism.

With a few exceptions of well-defined conditions that adhere to specific causal mechanisms, in all other health conditions, even when a primary causal agent is determined, there are secondary, tertiary factors whose significance may vary dramatically from one case to another.

Health is an entire universe full of intricate interrelations and not a medical algebra. Adding and subtracting, multiplying and dividing does not always suffice to provide us with a trustworthy medical outcome.

But once again we fall victims to overspecializing, oversimplifying or overgeneralizing. And we are certainly falling victims to our own gullibility, greed and irrationalism.

Statins. The hit cholesterol-lowering drugs that are believed to lower heart disease risks have been characterized as wonder-drugs. Statins have become an ever-expanding medical trend. To expand the market, the acceptable cholesterol limits are lowered. And statin sales move up. In 2004 statin sales reached $15 billion.[40] And that wasn't enough. In 2008 a huge study involving more than 18,000 healthy subjects, the so-called Jupiter study, concluded that statin use lowers heart disease risks even in recipients with normal cholesterol levels.[41] With just one big study the road to a new and huge target group for statin sales is paved. Statin use has been even recommended by the prestigious American Academy of Pediatrics for high risk profiled children of as young as 8 years old. Voila, one prestigious recommendation, another one huge target group for drug sales. Again it works like a charm. Statins work miracles intended not necessarily to those who buy and consume them, but definitely so to those who produce and sell them. Statins are almost a dream come true for Big Pharma; they almost realize former Merck's CEO Henry Gadsden's vision of selling drugs to healthy people, of maximizing drug target groups and companies' profits. "I would have preferred Merck to be more like the chewing-gum manufacturer Wrigley, because then Merck would be able to "sell to everyone."[42] That's what the man actually said back then, and now statins are close to achieving a historical victory over the unmedicated, the "natural" state of health. And if statins achieve this breakthrough it will be because of their illusive application. Statins do not treat actual diseases. They "lower risks", and risks are not as tangible as real diseases nor are they usually of an urgent nature, nor can be easily assessed. Statins can be taken for life to prevent conditions that their user may never develop even without statin use. Statins tend now to become a cultural phenomenon, a lasting, persisting and widespread medical fashion and habit like aspirin, painkillers and diet pills.

But, statins are drugs. The fact remains that all chemical substances are toxic and their benefit/risk profile reverses after they exceed a specific dosage threshold and they become toxic or adverse to health. Even oxygen and water in extremely highly dosages can be hazardous, even deadly. Chemical compounds even more so. Besides that, drugs additionally cause side effects. Statins have been loosely associated with memory loss.[43] And this is just a hint of possible side effects related to medications taken for life. But while side effect triggering mechanisms are not explored thoroughly, improbable biochemical correlations and therapeutic claims are made in relation to benefits from statin use.

One good example of an empirical and shallow statin benefit allegation can be found in a rather recent issue of the *Archives of Ophthalmology*. The article states – "The long term use of statins to control hypercholesterolemia – one of the leading cause of blindness among people older than 63. This information was reproduced in "Medical Briefs".[44] Medical Briefs summed up the analysis of the researchers by saying, "The use of statins for 24 months or more was associated with a significant reduction in risk for glaucoma. The use of non-statin cholesterol-lowering medications was also associated with a significantly reduced risk for glaucoma." The article further promoted the long-term use of statins by stating, "the results indicate the intriguing possibility that long-term oral statins may reduce risk of open-angle glaucoma, particularly among those with cardiovascular and lipid diseases."

Is this twisted science or just a fallacy or something based on half truths? Let's examine the issue closely. In Medical Briefs, there is no caution on the long-term use of statins or other cholesterol-lowering drugs or if they also lower the natural coenzyme Q10 production in the body that could precipitate a health problem or disruption in glycolysis. We know that the more LDL-cholesterol in the blood, the greater is the risk of heart disease. The link between high LDL and glaucoma are not explained in Medical Briefs. The cause of glaucoma is not known, but many doctors believe it is related to poor blood flow to the optic nerve. Glaucoma is more common in those who have a history of vascular disease.

Glaucoma actually represents many different diseases, affecting all age groups from newborns to the elderly. It can be very painful, or can progress without any symptoms. Glaucoma is a major cause of irreversible blindness. Glaucoma is often associated with high pressure in the eyes, however, a high percentage of people with glaucoma have normal or even low pressure. Ultimately, the final cause of vision loss in each type of glaucoma is an inability to get the needed nutrients to the cells of the retina and optic nerve, as well as to remove metabolic wastes and any other toxins that may be present in these tissues of the central nervous system and drug treatment for hypertension can increase glaucoma damage. So, what is the link between glaucoma, cardiovascular disease and drugs used to treat cardio-vascular disease?

The answer may lie in the fact that macula degeneration, cataract, glaucoma and cardiovascular disease are caused by allergens from protozoa and/or excess free radicals or associated with the lowering of the blood antioxidant levels with increasing age. Obese people and people with diabetes have relatively more free radicals in their bodies. Free radicals cause protein damage. If proteins in the lens of the eye are damaged by free radicals, the damaged proteins form cross links that reduce the amount of light entering the eye and vision is also affected if proteins found in the capillaries of the eye is damaged by free radicals; they may react with sugars in the blood and may get attached to the capillary walls and reduce blood flow. Similarly, oxidized LDL may get deposited in the capillaries of the eye and reduce blood flow. Reduced blood flow will only aid the degenerative process in the affected areas of the eye. Most allopathic drugs generate free radicals and the drugs used to treat cardiovascular disease add to the excess free radical population in the body of people with cardiovascular disease and help in the progression of glaucoma (and other conditions).

So, the observation of researchers in the article in the Archives of Ophthalmology is based on the fact that reduced LDL levels means a lower risk of oxidized LDL being deposited in the capillaries of the eyes. That means a proper scientific conclusion ought to be stated in terms of the benefits of a high HDL/LDL ratio with a low LDL level and promoting a diet rich in antioxidants. The reduced risk of glaucoma is therefore due to a lower risk of oxidized LDL (by lowering it) and it should not be said that "the long term use of statins may reduce the risk of glaucoma."

Scientific temper must attempt to unravel the truth for the actual benefit of humanity and human health. Science must never be twisted to promote the revenues of corporations that sell drugs such that their bottom line improves at the expense of human health. Hence, medical literature must be continually scrutinized.

Statins allegedly reduce heart disease risks. But so does exercise,[45] which additionally improves total lipoprotein profile,[46] offering a more thorough cardiovascular disease preventive mechanism. Consumption of omega-3 fatty acids from seafood or supplements benefits people at risk for coronary heart disease.[47]

It is clear that there is a multitude of preventive strategies against heart disease. But we stick to the more burdening one to individual and public health: Statins. Are we too lazy or too busy to be fit? Are we too busy or too lazy to have a prudent diet? Are we too greedy to let go of the billions of dollars worth trade of statins? Are we too gullible to think on our own? Are we too specialized to understand that usually a focal intervention in a huge biochemical and psychological chain of events is not enough to do the trick? Are we too simple-minded to understand that there are no magic pills? Off course we are. All of the afore-mentioned are true. And the dots, when connected, do not only reveal things about medicine but depict the ugly side of our civilization more precisely. They make up a business culture. Our culture now comprises of junk food, empty calories, synthetic molecules such as trans-fatty acids and aspartame, the sofa mentality and a more sedentary lifestyle, the junk science culture, the magic bullet superstition and the myth of drugs as part of a curative science that constantly derides the use of natural biomolecules whether produced in the body as part of healthy biochemistry or in plants that are part of healthy diet in therapy. Our once vibrant and almost rational culture has become a technomagical civilization which day by day sinks deeper into its own eccentric lifestyle, into the inertness of experts and authorities' reassurances and into a slowly decaying health state. We are clearly out of balance.

So, it is always about balance, fine tuning. It is about walking the thin line between too much and too little, it is about the equilibrium, it is about the principle of life called homeostasis. In the human body, the biological system in the healthy state manages its balance or equilibrium through its natural steroids and its natural antioxidant system that form part of its regulatory mechanisms. Drug pushers and synthetic vitamin pushers alike create a health-related market that is neither a healthy market nor a market for health.

In the supplement and diet market, there exists a very fertile soil for magic pills to pop up. Fen-phen was another diet messiah. And like most self-proclaimed messiahs, it turned out to be a catastrophe.

### c) Why doctors will give you only half-truths about...
### The Weak Science of Chemically-induced Weight Loss
Slimmer, sexier, more successful in one's professional and personal life: who could honestly resist such an offer? Especially when it demands of you nothing more than consuming systematically a chemical product, a pill? It sounds too good to be true. And to be completely honest, it is too good to be true, in fact it is

not true and to make things even worse it can turn out to be disastrous.

We have lived in a culture of image, not reason. Everything appears to be possible when most of the time it is not. Impressions and not judgment govern our lives. We live under the impression that movie stars, models, pop idols are self-evidently thin and sexy. We tend to think that there is no personal effort involved in their almost-perfect looks. So we tend to conclude that we can also effortlessly look like them.

Our gullibility, our improvidence and our greed has led to the creation of a need and a demand: we want to be transformed into impeccable caricatures. And the industry genies would answer our prayers.

We have misdirected and distorted our inner dream machine to accept and produce junk and plastic. But our psyche refused to conform to its industrialization, separated as it was from our idle omnivorous bodies that refused to move to perform any action to fulfill their real purposes and to meet their real needs.

The industry simply didn't care for our condition and our plight. It dashed forward and using bad science it tried to seize the moment and capitalize on our weakness, our misunder-standing of the real inner and outer world, on our divorce from our souls and the surrounding reality, our being kept hostages by an ideal virtuality and artificiality.

The industry encouraged by our cheap dreams made promises it couldn't possibly keep: Wanna look thin? Forget personal effort. Take this magic pill and you, frog, will be trans-formed into prince charming.

There were many chemical nominees claiming they could do wonders for our silhouette. During the nineties, one of them prevailed and led to a public health calamity.

It was called Fen-phen. Its predecessor was fenfluramine. Fenfluramine would meddle with the body's serotonin, increasing serotonin levels in the organism thus leading to a feeling of satiation. Unfortunately, even appetite is a complex phenomenon, involving not only somatic but also psychological and even symbolic factors, as any other human desire. A chemical switch could never possibly be up to the task of precise behavioral modulation. Moreover, as serotonin is involved in many and complex neural functions, the drug's side effects were respectively numerous and complex. As the former FDA drug reviewer Dr. Leo Lutwak stated, "Pondimin (fenflouramine) was not widely used. It just didn't make people feel that good... To this day, I remain concerned about the neuropsychiatric side effects – mood changes, memory loss, and so on. I don't think it ever has been fully explored."[48]

The serotonin version of the one factor-one behavior pattern supposition would be later employed by psychiatry to produce another monument of junk science, the use of SSRIs in the treatment of depression as we will see in the corresponding chapter.

So the industry gurus thought: OK, we got fenfluramine and it doesn't work all that well but at least we have a ridiculous medical supposition to pursue it commercially. But what to do with the pestering side effects?

Eureka! We blend it with something that will slim down fenfluramine's side effects; we combine it with the stimulant phentermine. Behold: a miraculous diet pill, Fen-phen was born.

The pharmaceutical commercial plots were designed at an era when obesity was beginning to get medicalized, that is, being treated not as a symptom of other underlying original causes but rather as an autonomous sickness, a trend that has developed also in blood pressure and cholesterol blood levels: symptoms are selectively isolated from the great picture of health and sickness and treated as autonomous diseases, leaving thus the underlying causes untreated. And this deliberate short-sightedness would turn out to be catastrophic.

With obesity disassociated from its real causes and Fen-phen dissociated from its mode of action and possible side effects, Americans would dash by the thousands to their doctors and pharmacies to ensure their access to the wonder drug.

Kate Cohen describes competently the Fen-phen frenzy:

"What was particularly shocking to me was that on the heels of reporting that this drug caused a fatal, incurable disease in Europe, the company was planning to put it on the American marketplace," says Dr. Stuart Rich, who co-authored the pulmonary hypertension study. Despite testimony from Dr. Rich and the opinions of two experts on neurotoxicity, the FDA approved dexfenfluramine in April 1996. "Just three months after the introduction of Redux, doctors are writing 85,000 prescriptions a week," Time Magazine reported in a cover story titled "The New Miracle Drug?"

Neurotoxicity was a foreseen and predictable possible side effect. What was not expected was the effect the "appetite suppressant" drug would have on heart valve cells. How could they predict it? The industry is too busy and overzealous trying to find the slightest theoretical beneficial correlation between chemical substances and biological mechanisms to pay any attention to or explore the full spectrum of interaction between substances and organisms.

This research cursoriness combined with the customers' gullibility, wishful thinking and the luck of meticulousness exhibited by the authorities in charge, led thousands of Fen-phen users to develop heart valve disease and pulmonary hypertension. Under the pressure exerted by this public health disaster, the FDA was forced to withdraw the hazardous drug that was once proclaimed to be an innocent miracle worker. But the damage continued long after the medication ceased. According to a study the damage on the heart valve was ongoing even after the discontinuation of the "treatment". In addition a lot of Fen-phen victims needed surgical operations and subsequent medications. Not only did the diet pill lead to numerable human tragedies thus but it raised public health costs as well. This is the world of the illustrious drugs, of lustrous dreams and disastrous public health decisions.

In most of the cases, obesity is not even about a disease, let alone a symptom. It is about a human body, mind and soul. A human creature. When comfortable with his body and life, obesity is not even a problem for the obese, let alone a medical condition. In these cases obesity appears to be a choice, an embodiment of plentitude though it still holds the potential to lead to medical complications. When the obese is not happy with his condition, then we are facing the consequences of people living in a prison, devoid of sensory and emotional stimuli. Only dreams of a better, fuller life are allowed in the everyday life's prison and even dreams are corrected, distorted and directed towards consumption. We have to assume full responsibility for our existence and well-being. It is our job to make promises we can keep and get us to the promised land, the one we are going to build. You don't like being fat? Sweat it off and eat a prudent diet. This is the hard way, this is the only way. No one can safely transform you if you don't involve yourself in personal change. It sounds hard and half as attractive as a miracle drug, but it is worth its while. And it is safe. And reversionary. And healthy. And rewarding.

Some thousand years, the Greek hero Hercules stood in a crossroads. One road, the easy one, was the road of malice. The other, the hard one, was the one of virtue. He took the painstaking one and became a hero to be remembered for thousands of years to come. We as a civilization are choosing the easy road. But we constantly carry the crossroads inside of us. We can always become our own personal hero and beat that which is beating us. And it is beating us badly right now.

A diet pill that destroyed the health of thousands of unsuspecting human beings. And in another pharmaceutical crime against humanity, a pill for morning sickness, thalidomide, that cursed millions of babies with phocomelia and other serious birth defects.

We supposedly have strict science, and strict scientific and government supervising mechanisms, and institutions that supposedly guarantee our safety. Still, public health disasters frequently occur. What is going on? Have we been deceived?

**d)** *Why doctors will give you only half-truths about...*
**Drug Safety and Efficacy**

Fen-phen and the likes of it were not a unique phenomenon. Dozens of diet pills are sold over the counter, creating the delusion that there is an easy, technomagical way to evade personal responsibilities and get where you want to go instantly and effortlessly. This junk food perception appears to have affected with laziness and casualness not only the medical customers but also the drug manufacturers. According to WHO's 2008 *"Consolidated List of Products whose Consumption and/or Sale have been Banned, Withdrawn, Severely Restricted or Not Approved by Governments"*, a total of 27 governments took regulatory actions on 88 drugs![49] This is not a number to be taken lightly. Some of these drugs have been blockbusters or at least used often in common medical practice for years or even decades, drugs like the analgesics-antipyretics Nimesulide and Metamizole sodium, the cough-suppressant Clobutinol, the "mood stabilizers" Carbamazepine and Lamotrigine, the anti-bedwetting Desmopressin nasal sprays, the anti-asthmatic Ephedrine, the anti-acne Isotretinoin, the local anesthetic and anti-arrhythmic Lidocaine, the anti-lice and anti-scabies Lindane, the non-steroidal anti-inflammatory Lumiracoxib, Piroxicam, Valdecoxib, the anxiolytic Meprobamate, the antiemetics Metoclopramide and Trimethobenzamide, the "anti-HIV" Nevirapine, the "anti-ADHD" Pemoline, the anti-Parkinson's D.

Pergolide, the anorectic, anti-obesity Rimonabant, the anti-diabetic Rosiglitazone, the antipsychotic Thioridazine. An entire class of drugs, the COX-2 selective inhibitors came under fire. But they were originally approved, weren't they, and their side effects could have been anticipated due to their specific modus operandi. From cough to vomit, from nocturnal leg cramps to bedwetting, from acne to Attention Deficit Hyperkinetic Disorder, from nausea to pain, most of the conditions that the regulated drugs were prescribed for are common and not life-threatening. That means that the risk/benefit ratio should have been better evaluated and the side effects should have been detected much earlier, not after years or decades of extensive use. Some of these drugs were not only dangerous but also "non efficacious", in other words useless, or of no proven therapeutic value. But wait! They successfully completed their clinical trials, were deemed both safe and efficient and after years of circulating in the general populace scientists, authorities and companies simply decide to change their minds over them? So, can anyone oblige us and tell us, what the blip went wrong? Was it perhaps that the whimsical clinical trials goddesses, Efficacy and Safety, made up their minds? Are there data goblins eating away the reliability of the clinical trial tree? Granted, if we want to have drugs out there, we cannot afford to wait for the full spectrum of a drug's actions and interactions to manifest itself nor can we test a drug on the entire population of the earth to draw safe conclusions. On the other hand, drug manufacturers spend their R&D disproportionately on finding a clever drug mechanism that will intercept a health condition benefiting thus the patient and they tend to ignore how and when the same mechanism will interact with other mechanisms in the body, creating side effects. We are not talking about pure science here, we are talking mostly about profit-motivated scientists and entrepreneurs. Research gets often blinded by greed and ambition.

Granted, some things will escape both researchers' and

authorities' attention. But when obvious side effects are ignored or underreported by drug recipients due to blind faith in medicine and medical illiteracy, or due to Big Pharma cover-ups and smokescreens, when the "Ooops, I did it again" effect is dominant, then, there is no doubt, something is rotten in the state of Drugmark. How can hepatotoxicity, a much anticipated and feared side effect, escape them; how can it disguise itself and hide from the expert eyesight of researchers? And why does it take authorities years and some times decades to decide that a drug was, from the very beginning, dangerous and potentially deadly? Why does there have to be dozens of reported side effect cases stacked before regulatory actions are taken? Isn't a single death attributable to a drug a strong indicator of lethality on a larger scale? Authorities have been systematically overhyping sporadic cases of deaths attributable to "novel epidemics" and rogue viral strains and almost instantly raise public health preparedness to Alarm Level. Hardly ever do they exhibit such a sensitivity and sound the alert about rogue drugs until drug-induced death is irrefutable and widespread.

Let us not forget the tragic example of Thalidomide, given to pregnant women to relieve morning sickness, the gruesome drug that spawned an entire generation of children with phocomelia and turned thousands of babies into living (or long gone) monuments of medical oversight, greed and arrogance. Who will be able to compensate these wonderful and dignified people and their families for the pain of pharmaceutical mutilation and incapacitation?

We have already exhibited that double-blind clinical trials are unreliable by definition due to the extent and variability of the placebo phenomenon. Now add to this fundamental unrelia-bility bad clinical trial designing, unreliable clinical trial statis-tical processing and, on top of all that, insufficient evaluation by the appointed officials or scientific corpuses with a twist of external pressures and influences, including mutual interests or contrasts of interests, a bit of corruption and direct or indirect bribery from time to time, well, there you have it: something rotten in the state of drug evaluation. Something rotten and potentially deadly.

The drug evaluation system has a lot of vulnerabilities. Some of them are expected, some are not. Some of them are accepted, others are definitely not. A vulnerable drug evaluation system makes us, the citizens of the world and the final recipients of a drug, equally vulnerable. It also renders the medical system weak. It is an innate sickness of a system that was originally invented, designed and evolved in order to fight sickness. This is only one oxymoron of the many that are innate in Pulp Medicine. Until this antisocial and anti-scientific infection is fought competently, no cure will be competently free of doubt.

## Chapter 2

# Cancer

*a) Why doctors will give you only half-truths about...*
**The War on Cancer**
We pretty much all know of Hamlet, one of the greatest heroes global theater has ever produced, a man who had to face terrible dilemmas in life and death. Now, if Hamlet was a modern doctor or a medical scientist his ruminations might have been slightly different. If I am given the poetic license, Dr. Hamlet's soliloquy might sound something like this:

> To treat, or not to treat: that is the question:
> Whether 'tis nobler in the mind to suffer
> The slings and arrows of outrageous *medicine*,
> Or to take arms against a sea of troubles,
> And by opposing end them

The slings and arrows of outrageous medicine. Despite the outrageous technological advance, modern medicine more often than not uses slings and arrows to defend both life and itself. Medicine has partly remained a *craft*, in which one man's skills can determine another one's life or death.

But let's not do modern medicine such a great injustice. M.M. is not contented to slings and arrows nor only to sticks and stones. In the great war theaters of health, such as cancer and AIDS, medicine, more often than not, uses napalms and other weapons of mass cell destruction. The enemy has to be crushed, annihilated. What if along with the enemy cells entire populations of healthy unarmed cells are harmed? No, it is not a tragedy nor a massacre. It is called collateral damage.

We know of cancer cells, how they work, what they do, how they disguise themselves from life and death. What we don't know is cancer itself. We tend to think of cancers as focal points that are unfit cells which turn into gangsters and take over the 'cellhood'. We send in our chemical troops to suppress the insurrection before it gets out of hand. But we hardly ever think: What turns a person or a cell into an 'unfit'? What makes a person or a cell turn against his own kin?

Modern medical science has failed to gear itself to look into the underlying causes, and remains content with treating the symptoms. As usual, the focus is the commercial angle – produce a drug that can get an approval for use in treatment. It is the business of managing treatments and patents and how they impact the current bottom line and business in the future.

The approach of facing force and violence with even greater force or violence has historically failed. It only transposes the problem to the future. But the problem usually remains, hibernated or simply hidden, waiting for the ripe conditions to reveal itself. The best way to confront superiority of forces is guerilla warfare. And that's what diseases also do under pressure.

The prominent dogma of cancer treatment has not been productive nor resourceful. Although, we now have more drugs and more treatments and better diagnostic tools, things are definitely not looking that great for the cancer patient, especially those past the third stage. For those receiving treatments for the early stages, there is good hope for many but it may just be a case of remission. Usually, little or nothing is done during the remission phase to detox the toxic chemo-drugs or to remove the oxidative stress and to organize a change in the diet to include a range of dietary antioxidants. And, unfortunately, not enough is being done in preventive medicine to reduce the risks to cancer and reduce the incidence of the various cancers based on diet.

In a 2005 report it was estimated that in 30 years time, the incidence of breast and lung cancer had doubled.[50]

According to a 2003 WHO report, *"Global cancer could increase by 50% to a 15 million by 2020."*[51]

Things are definitely not looking good. One easy to grasp aspect of the cancer increase conundrum is without a doubt the aging of the global population. The longer the organism lives the more possible it is to develop a type of cancer during its lifespan. The Population Division of the UN Department of Economic and Social Affairs, in 2002, issued a report that reached to some ominous conclusions. According to the report:

Population aging is unprecedented, without parallel in human history—and the twenty-first century will witness even more rapid aging than did the century just past.

Population aging is enduring: we will not return to the young populations that our ancestors knew.

Population aging has profound implications for many facets of human life."[52]

There is no doubt that a small percentage of cancer incidence increase is due to the population aging phenomenon. Nevertheless it is impossible to attribute it entirely to humanity growing older. Because the increase in cancer incidence involves as well the youthful part of the general population. The International Agency for Research on Cancer reported that in Europe cancer rates have been increasing by around 1% annually for children, and 1.5% annually for adolescents from the 1970s to the 1990s. This is a pattern that concerns not only Europe but the entirety of the developed world.[53] We are losing the war and we are losing it so hard that we are forced to come to terms with the enemy: *"New drugs will not necessarily eradicate tumors, but when used in combination with other agents may turn many cases of rapidly fatal cancer into 'manageable' chronic illness,"* Bernard Stewart, Director of Cancer Services admits.[54] Another admission of defeat comes from *Scientific American*:

Perhaps, as safe oral antiangiogenic drugs are developed and become available, cancer patients will be able to take "a pill a day to keep the cancer away". If so, forms of cancer that are currently untreatable will be reduced to chronic health problems similar to hypertension or diabetes, and many more people will be able to live long satisfying lives.[55]

So what is actually happening?

This is a tough question to answer. There are thousands of cancer risk factors. Among them are behavioral patterns that are repeatedly met in the developed world, "lifestyle" patterns. According to the WHO: *"The Western lifestyle is characterized by a highly caloric diet, rich in fat, refined carbohydrates and animal protein, combined with low physical activity, resulting in an overall energy imbalance."*[56] Despite the recognition of an unhealthy lifestyle that facilitates cancer development, the WHO anticancer strategies are not oriented towards a healthier lifestyle but rather towards early diagnostic and treatment strategies, that is, towards strategies that intervene after the onset of cancer and are costly either for the individual or for the med care system and therefore for the society in total. So, once again, in cancer, disease-oriented and not health-oriented strategies are promoted and employed. It must be understood that health and disease exist in the continuum of Life. The more cornered or neglected health is the more room there is for sickness to expand.

Sharon Begley described accurately this lack of vision and prudence that runs through the Cancer Research Foundation from its early days in her excellent analysis in Newsweek titled *"We fought cancer... and cancer won"*. For Begley, a great opportunity was missed regarding

... the use of natural compounds and nondrug interventions such as stress reduction to keep the microenvironment inhospitable to cancer... "Funding has gone to easier areas to research, like whether a drug can prevent cancer recurrence," says Lorenzo Cohen, who runs the integrative care center at M.D. Anderson. That's simpler to study, he points out, than whether a complicated mix of diet, exercise and stress reduction techniques can keep the micro-environment hostile to cancer.

Begley ponders that now is the

... time to consider the missed opportunities of the first 37 years of the war on cancer. Surely the greatest is prevention. Nixon never used the word; he exhorted scientists only to find a cure. Partly as a result, the huge majority of funding for cancer has gone into the search for ways to eradicate malignant cells rather than to keep normal cells from becoming malignant in the first place. "The funding people are interested in the magic-bullet research because that's what brings the dollars in," says oncologist Anthony Back, of the Hutch. "It's not as sexy to look at whether broccoli sprouts prevent colon cancer. A reviewer looks at that and asks, 'How would you ever get that to work?' "And besides, broccoli can't be patented, so without the potential payoff of a billion-dollar drug there is less incentive to discover how cancer can be prevented.[57]

One could say that the great strategic fallacies embarked under the Nixon administration and the declaration of the war on cancer. It was one of the many wars to follow: the war on drugs, the war on science, the war on terror. A masculine, aggressive, warlike approach, bent on leveling the "enemy" by all means. Historically, such approaches are hardly ever effective. The "threat" is usually dealt with for the short term, it lays low for the period of time when the balance of power does not favor it, only to re-emerge battle hardened and more adaptive and flexible in the long term.

Another excellent commentator on the war on cancer and the reasons why it is failing is Clifton Leaf. Clifton is much more than an objective commentator or a knowledgeable scientific reporter or just an impartial journalist. He is a cancer survivor, a former kid who fought the battle of his life in his teens and lived to tell the story. Clifton delivers us his critique on the Cancer Research Foundation after conversing with leading cancer researchers:

> ...Yet virtually all these experts offered testimony that, when taken together, describes a dysfunctional "cancer culture" – a groupthink that pushes tens of thousands of physicians and scientists toward the goal of finding the tiniest improvements in treatment rather than genuine breakthroughs; that fosters isolated (and redundant) problem solving instead of cooper-ation; and rewards academic achievement and publication over all else.

> At each step along the way from basic science to patient bedside, investigators rely on models that are consistently lousy at predicting success – to the point where hundreds of cancer drugs are thrust into the pipeline, and many are approved by the FDA, even though their proven "activity" has little to do with curing cancer.

> "It's like a Greek tragedy," observes Andy Grove, the chairman of Intel and a prostate-cancer survivor, who for years has tried to shake this cultural mindset as a member of several cancer advisory groups. "Everybody plays his individual part to perfection, everybody does what's right by his own life, and the total just doesn't work."

> Tragedy, unfortunately, is the perfect word for it. Heroic figures battling forces greater than themselves. Needless death and destruction. But unlike Greek tragedy, where the Fates predetermine the outcome, the nation's cancer crusade

didn't have to play out this way. And it doesn't have to stay this way.[58]

Overspecialization, with the good it did for research by assigning different and discrete roles to researchers, brought about an unnecessary evil. The specialists were so focused in their research object that they became myopic and started to overlook the bigger picture. Leaf characteristically emphasized that in 2003, of the 8900 grant proposals awarded by the NCI, 92% of them didn't even mention the word metastasis. And metastasis is ultimately crucial for the survival and well-being of the cancer patient.

It is all about focus. Focused biochemistry, obsessed with finding one particular tiny particle, or tiny receptor. It is all about Micro-science and micro-scientists. But micro means small and sometimes to solve a problem that you just can't get around, you have to think big, you have to think outside of the box, think and process not only isolated data but mostly correlations and integrations.

Leaf comments with the wisdom of a scientific Methuselah on this micro-science of our times:

Yet somehow, along the way, something important has gotten lost. The search for knowledge has become an end unto itself rather than the means to an end. And the research has become increasingly narrow, so much so that physician-scientists who want to think systemically about cancer or the organism as a whole – or who might have completely new approaches – often can't get funding [59]

It is so obvious by now. We have to think as a whole, act as a whole and treat the organism as a whole. The Lego science, the brick by brick science has not been able to treat cancer.

Cancer, despite the hysteric declarations against it, is not an invader from outer space. Carcinogenesis is not an anomaly; in a way, carcinogenesis is quite natural. Every day in each and every one of us cancer cells are given birth to but are arrested early by our immune system. Carcinogenesis turns to cancer only when cell populations have lost their vigor, only when imbalances allow it to do so.

So, with some exceptions, cancer is not only about how it is created. It is more about the general condition of the organism and the immune system.

The Cancer Research Foundation, though not governed by systemic perceptions, fell easily into the same systemic errors that seem to be idiomatic of modern medicine. At the same time that it was narrowed by overspecialization, it was stretched beyond its scope by overgeneralization.

The perception of one drug, one magic bullet to treat all cancers, of the marvel drug, reveals an underlying misconception of the "One Cancer for All and One Treatment for All Cancers" mentality. And though hardly any cancer specialist or health expert will agree to the notion of the one cancer, the Cancer Research Foundation seems to informally validate the one cancer dogma.

Overspecialization that tends to overlook the greater picture, overgeneralization that invents the median man and the three musketeers-like "one for all and all for one" cancer research culture are constantly jeopardizing research, public health and global economy.

And cancer responds to the challenges, declaring pompously: "I am legion, for I am many."

This is a reality that is being widely recognized by now. But a cumbersome state and medical bureaucracy fails to keep up with the advancements in the perceptions of cancer and entraps novelty and innovation in an obsolete and failed modus operandi.

Many cancers, many cancer patients, many cancer strategies,

all equal and all different. That is the way to go. A personalized medicine, a democratic medicine that recognizes and respects individuality, not the Big Brother medicine, nor the Big Pharma medicine, not the communist medicine, the populist medicine, the Pulp Medicine that embraces everyone with uniform solutions. They obviously don't work. They are not designed or meant for you. They address the invented average guy. Granted, the average guy may have the best medicine possible. The only problem is that the average blob does not exist. And the rest of us, that is, all of us, are completely disregarded by Pulp Med.

The need for diverse and versatile cancer solutions has been repeatedly recognized and designated. It has become evident by now that this is the way to go.

Sharon Begley characteristically cites Roy Herbst: *"The hope is to match tumor type to drug… we need to make the next leap, getting the right drug to the right patient."*[60]

And Clifton Leaf cites Elli Lilly's Homer Pearce:

I think everyone believes that at the end of the day, cancer is going to be treated with multiple targeted agents – maybe in combination with traditional chemotherapy drugs, maybe not. Because that's where the biology is leading us, it's a future that we have to embrace – though it will definitely require different models of cooperation.[61]

A step towards this direction, a multiple and personalized cancer strategy seems, to already have been achieved. The wheel seems to turn, slowly, painstakingly; still, it is turning a bit.

An experimental drug, olaparib, showed really promising results when tested on 19 patients with advanced breast, ovarian and prostate cancer. The drug, belonging to the class of parp inhibitors, draws its anticancerous properties from a notion called synthetic lethality and is so far applicable to patients with mutations in their BRCA1 and BRCA2 genes. BRCA1 and BRCA2 belong to a class of genes called "tumor suppressors" and are involved in the multifactorial DNA repair mechanism.[62] The patients that underwent the therapy showed impressive therapeutic results or at least had their cancers controlled without the side effects of conventional chemotherapy.[63] Although, at the present stage of development, only the few cancer patients with BRCA1 and BRCA2 mutations may benefit from this tailored drug, for them, olaparib might make all the difference in the world.

Out there, in the Great Cosmos of cancer research, there are a lot of great opportunities to outsmart cancer and not just bomb it as it has been traditionally done so far. Sharon Begley commenting on the missed opportunity involving the environment around a tumor cell quotes MIT's Robert Weinberg: "We used to focus on cancer cells with the idea that they were master of their own destiny." "By studying genes inside the cell we thought we could understand what was going on. But now [we know] that many tumors are governed by the signals they receive from outside"—from inflammatory cells, cells of the immune system and others. "It's the interaction of signals inside and outside the tumor that creates aggressiveness and metastasis."

And Genentech got that signal, the SOS that the sinking, therapeutically, armada of cancer research was sending out. And it responded with bevacizumab (trade name Avastin), a monoclonal antibody that inhibits the formation of new vessels by targeting and inhibiting Vascular Endothelial Growth Factor (VEGF), thus restricting tumor angiogenesis and metastasis.[64] And though Avastin has serious side effects, aggressively inhibits basic life functions, is expensive and may not be the miracle worker it was originally professed to be, it is thought a welcome therapeutic alternative, one more tool at the disposal of the practitioner and patient to use at their will.

A similar approach is being investigated by Exelixis, with its

Xl series of vaccines that target the MET and VEGFR2 receptors, potentially blocking or restraining tumoral invasive and angiogenic mechanisms.

And Gern explores another mechanism that holds perhaps an even greater potential, that of telomerase, an enzyme that plays a crucial role in aging in general and in cell line immortality. But perhaps, the great promise lies elsewhere, in the unexplored and unexploited vastness of our immune system. The immune system along with the nerve system are designed to interact with the vastness of the universe outside of us. By definition and by far they are the two most complex systems of evolved organisms, tending to the survival and adaptation of the organism to an ever changing and unpredictable environment. And judging from the outcome, us, the human species surviving and creating our own environments, they are doing an excellent job. Sometimes, they even work miracles.

Miracles like spontaneous remission. Many baffled practitioners and elated patients have witnessed tumors shrink to inexistence for no known reason. It is "either divine intervention or the immune system," confesses Jedd D. Wolchok, an oncologist at New York's Memorial Sloan-Kettering Cancer Center.[65]

Wolchok, obviously being able to mount immune responses easier than divine intervention, used ipilimumab, a monoclonal antibody expected to work as switch on for immune response to treat a lung cancer patient. And it worked. The patient's lung tumors shrunk. But when ipilimumab was put under the spotlight of clinical trials it failed to achieve the excellent performances that were expected of it. In one of the three related studies the primary endpoint was not met: less than 10% of the subjects' cancers responded to the therapy.[66] So what? If you asked a terminal cancer patient whether he would choose not a 10%, not even 1% but a 0.0001% chance of being cured over death, what would he actually choose? The Pulp Medicine, the bigger is better med and the ever-growing medical bureaucracy is depriving people of their essential rights to hope and heal. It is not only about quantity. Sometimes it is about quality, given that the quality exists even in one out of a million cases.

Immune therapy approaches have been tried since the early days of cancer research, but after interleukin-2 failed to become the cancer messiah they were pretty much abandoned. The killing techniques were preferred and it was exactly that strategy that led us to this lengthy and failing military campaign against cancer. Instead of tightening or relaxing the safety valves of our immune system, instead of encouraging it and enabling it, we chose to just bomb everything that looked like a threat with weapons of mass cellular destruction.

Strange as it may seem, a successful immune cancer strategy is not all about power. It is more about education. It is about educating our immune system to recognize friend from foe, excess from lack, too much from too little, overexposure from deficiency, balance from imbalance.

And this is exactly what Cassian Yee at the Fred Hutchinson Cancer Research Center did. He spotted white cells seemingly active against cancer from the blood of a 52-year-old man with advanced melanoma, pumped them out and copiously cultured them. He then re-injected them multiplied into the patients' blood stream to attack the cancer. What worked marvelously for one patient didn't work for 8 others. Robert Langreth in his magnificent piece "Cancer Miracles" quotes UCLA oncologist Antoni Ribas commenting on the whims of immune response: "It's the hallmark of immune therapy – it doesn't happen often, but once it happens, those patients live years."[67]

A similar approach of a tumor cell-specific autologous "vaccine" is reportedly followed by German biochemist H. Anthopoulos at his privately funded Clinical Biochemical Institute for Cell Biotechnology and Immunology.[68]

Following a similar rational, a small company named Dendreon developed an immunological "vaccine" for patients with advanced prostate cancer. In 2009 there were 192,280 new cases of prostate cancer in the US, with 27,360 people dying of it.[69] In advanced prostate cancer there are few available treatments and they are definitely not attractive. Dendreon came up with an elegant approach: sipuleucel-T (trade name Provenge). Provenge is not so much of a drug but rather a medical procedure. Autologous APC's (antigen presenting cells) are taken from patients' blood, co-cultured with a protein that contains prostatic acid phosphatase (PAP), an enzyme that can be found in 95% of prostate cancers. The PAP-informed APC's are then injected back to the patient.

Provenge has been shown to prolong survival of advanced prostate cancer patients, yet it was not approved by the FDA in 2007, a decision that fueled an anti-bureaucratic form of activism by family members who were helplessly watching their loved ones sitting on the death row of the metastatic prostate cancer prognosis.

And CEL-SCI Corporation is testing their promising multitasking immunostimulant, Multikine, which consists of a mixture of naturally occurring cytokines including interleukins, interferons, chemokines and colony-stimulating factors

Stephen Rosenberg, of the US National Cancer Institute team in Bethesda, is still another researcher that attempted to train the immune system against cancer. He took T-cells from malignant melanoma patients, used viruses as gene vectors to equip the T-cells with receptors so that they could recognize the melanoma and re-infused them into the patients to fight the melanoma. Eighteen months later, 2 out of 17 patients were rid of their cancers.[70] One small step for cancer, one giant leap for a cancer patient.

There is no doubt that there is a dysfunctional cancer culture out there. The survival of 1 out of 10 cancer patients is not worthwhile? What about the value of life? What about having the choice and the luxury of 100 more immune therapies and making wise decisions that will lead to the long-term survival of 9 out of 10 patients without the gruesome side effects of chemotherapy and radiation? What about taking the path less taken that will perhaps lead us to the promised land of effective cancer treatment?

Until now, the patient is perceived and treated as a weak-minded, obedient automaton and his only participation in the medical system is to comply with doctor's orders. He is not only held hostage by an inhuman medical system. He is in every possible sense a medical slave. It is time for the medical liberation.

Our fate, our own health lies in our hands. It is about us being knowledgeable, informed, confident. It is about us encouraging a research mentality that prefers versatility and abundance of therapeutic options over monolithic uniform solutions. It is ultimately about self-empowerment and education, it is about being informed and educated enough to be able to inform and educate our immune system to do the job for us. Things are more complex than we tend to think they are, and only when this wonderful complexity is understood and it begins to saturate us socially and scientifically, only then will we be able to understand the working simplicity beyond the striking complexity.

Thousands of years ago, a Greek epic poet wrote about the adventures of Ulysses. Ulysses was the one who in Iliad contrived of the Trojan horse to capture the great city of Troy, which resisted force alone. He is the one that escaped the cave of the Cyclops Polyphemus by blinding his only eye and exiting unnoticed tied to the undersides of his huge sheep. When asked of his name by Polyphemus, Ulysses misinformed him that his name was No One. So when the blinded Cyclops asked for help from his fellow Cyclops he was crying out, "No one has hurt me."

Now, almost 3000 years later, cancer research is as one-eyed as all Cyclops were and blinded as Polyphemus was by the stick of greed. When asked what is hurting us we answer "cancer" unaware of its true name. So many centuries of medical advances and yet cancer is toying with us like a microscopic Ulysses. We owe it to ourselves to be at least as smart as he was. It is time we revered educated scientists who possess a broader scope of things, scientists that might even have heart or read literature. The lab rats can only tell rat cancers. And rat cancers are so much easier to treat than human cancers. And that is because, we, as a species, are not made only of cells but of emotions and thoughts as well. It is time that cancer is addressed by people who understand that perplexity of sentient organisms and will get cancer's name for us. Its real name.

*b) Why doctors will give you only half-truths about...*
**Nature's Cancer Prevention – Vitamin B17**
Your oncologist may not tell you about the chemo paradox – that it does not kill cancer cells selectively while it kills young and healthy cells as well. Chemotherapy can also deplete minerals in your body while it can set up oxidative stress as well. He may not tell you the cause of the chronic inflammation that led to the formation of cancer cells or whether the cancer cells arose as a result of oxidative damage to the genetic molecules or how the chemo-drug acts against the cancer in the body. It is usually about the diagnosis and to proceed with the chemo-therapy and let you deal with the side effects of the therapy as they come. A good oncologist will discuss with you in as much detail as possible, but quite invariably few will ever mention non-toxic therapies or how increasing dietary intake of fat-soluble antioxidants, other than those foods that are rich in glutathione, can be integrated into conventional therapy.

You may have read about research in alternative medicine and the research involving edible substances that can disrupt the biochemical pathways in cancer cells or help to eliminate the charge on the cell membranes of cancer cells or inhibit their growth and inhibit tumor growth by preventing the formation of blood vessels in tumors or edible substances that can cause apoptosis of cancer cells.

"Numerous epidemiological studies revealed that high consumption of fruits, vegetables, and other plant products may reduce the incidence and development of colorectal cancer. Since colorectal cancers are difficult to treat with existing therapeutic modalities, identifying dietary phytochemicals that have anti-tumor activity and investigating their mechanisms of action may lead to significant advances in the prevention of human cancer. The monoterpenes, found in essential oils of citrus fruits, cherry, mint, and herbs, are non-nutritive dietary microconstituents mainly responsible for the distinctive fragrance of many plants."[71]

Geraniol and other monoterpenes found in essential oils of fruits and herbs have been suggested to represent a new class of agents for cancer chemoprevention. 400 µM of geraniol can cause a 70% inhibition of cell growth through inhibition of DNA synthesis without any signs of cytotoxicity or apoptosis. This inhibition in the growth of cancer cells by geraniol is due to a very significant decrease in ornithine decarboxylase activity, a key enzyme of polyamine biosynthesis, which is enhanced in cancer growth. Such decreases in ornithine decarboxylase activity also lead to a 40% reduction of the intracellular pool of putrescine. Geraniol also activated the intracellular catabolism of polyamines, indicated by enhanced polyamine acetylation. These observations indicate that geraniol metabolism appears to generate the antiproliferative properties in the targeted cancer cells.[72]

Recent studies have shown that monoterpenes exert anti-tumor activities and suggest that these components are a new class of cancer chemo-preventive agents.[73] Limonene, a main constituent of orange and citrus peel oils, has been reported to exert anti-tumor activity against mammary gland, lung, liver, stomach, and skin cancers in rodents.[74] Similarly, perillyl alcohol, an hydroxylated limonene analog, exhibits chemo-preventive activity against liver, mammary gland, pancreas, and colon cancers in rodents.[75] More recently, geraniol, an acyclic monoterpene alcohol found in lemongrass and aromatic herb oils, has been shown to exert in vitro and in vivo anti-tumor activity against murine leukemia, hepatoma, and melanoma cells.[76]

Pancreatic cancer, the fourth leading cause of cancer-associated mortality in the United States, usually presents in an advanced stage and is generally refractory to chemotherapy. As such, there is a great need for novel therapies for this disease. The naturally derived isoprenoids perillyl alcohol, farnesol, and geraniol have chemotherapeutic potential in pancreatic and other tumor types. Perillyl alcohol (POH), geraniol (GOH), and farnesol (FOH) are plant-derived isoprenoid compounds. Dietary sources of perillyl alcohol include cherries, spearmint, sage, and celery seeds. Examples of geraniol dietary sources include carrot, lemon, lime, nutmeg, orange, blueberry, and blackberry. Farnesol is found in lemongrass and chamomile. Certain plants, such as lavender, lemongrass, and rosemary, are sources for more than one isoprenoid. Each isoprenoid has chemo-preventive and therapeutic activity in a wide variety of in vitro and in vivo cancer models, including pancreatic cancer, for which there is little therapeutic success in the clinic. Perillyl alcohol and farnesol also tend to decrease DNA replication in pancreatic epithelial cell.[77]

Isoprenoids and terpenoids and triterpenoids from edible sources have been reported to have a number of molecular and cellular effects including reduction of blood glucose levels and inhibition of cholesterol biosynthesis, and these results are much better when the powders from these edible substances are then mixed with powders from plant sources that are rich in bioflavinoids and powders from plant parts especially that have anti-parasitic properties and consumed like tea, brewed with warm, not boiling water. In the future, integrative medicine may become more common especially in countries like India where such research is making important strides. These phytochemicals from food sources work well in the L-form biochemistry of the mammalian biological system and helps to promote healthy biochemical pathways, whereas the bioflavinoids and other natural antioxidants serve to remove or eliminate or otherwise reduce oxidative stress and help drive the L-form healthy biochemistry. The metabolism of such phytochemicals and natural antioxidants in normal and healthy cells is different from the metabolism of these biomolecules in cancer cells and such metabolism, having evolved over 900 million years, does not yield toxic molecules in healthy cells and their metabolism is either non-toxic or of very low toxicity. This difference in the metabolism of phytochemicals in healthy cells and cancer cells holds the key to safe therapy in the years ahead. Hence, a better understanding of cancer cell biochemistry and the metabolism of natural biomolecules will lead to more interesting therapies in cancer cells.

That leads to a need to discuss vitamin B17. Have you ever heard of vitamin B17? Maybe you have heard of its other name – Laetrile.

Americans cannot access vitamin B17 because the FDA took it off the market in the 1970s, and removed it from the B-Complex vitamins. It is unlawful for any health practitioner to administer this vitamin to patients. Apricot seeds are the best source for B17, but they have also been removed from the shelves of every health food store and natural market throughout the USA. Limited research has been conducted on vitamin B17 since 1977. Once it was banned, it was forgotten.

According to research from years ago, provided by nutritionists and medical scientists, vitamin B17 is a natural cyanide-containing compound that gives up its cyanide content only in the presence of a particular enzyme group called beta-glucosidase or -glucuronidase. Miraculously, this enzyme group is found almost exclusively in cancer cells. If found elsewhere in the body, it is accompanied by greater quantities of another enzyme, rhodanese, which has the ability to disable the cyanide and convert it into completely harmless substances. Cancer tissues do not have this protecting enzyme.

So, according to past scientific knowledge, cancer cells are faced with a double threat: the presence of one enzyme exposing them to cyanide, while the absence of another enzyme found in all other normal cells resulting in the cancer's failure to detoxify itself. Leave it to nature to provide a form of cyanide that can naturally destroy a cancer cell. The cancer cells that are unable to withstand the cyanide are destroyed, while the non-cancerous cells are not threatened by the cyanide, and, therefore, remain unharmed. Never underestimate the body's potential!

Vitamin B17 is found naturally in many foods. If you eat foods containing vitamin B17, your body will know what to do next. All other animals in nature instinctively do this. Consider it nature's cancer prevention. If only modern medicine would allow it.

San Francisco's Ernst T. Krebs, Sr., MD, discovered the healing qualities of vitamin B17 in 1923. His sons, Ernst T. Krebs, Jr., PhD, and Byron Krebs, MD, continued their father's research in 1952, refining Laetrile's (B17) nutritional qualities.

From their research, the Krebs believed cancer was not caused by an outside invading force but rather by malfunctions of the normal mechanics within the body itself. They identified cancer as a "deficiency disease". The body's malfunctions, according to their research, were the result of a deficiency of certain chemicals found in food, a deficiency of chemicals they specifically identified as vitamin B17, as well as a deficiency of enzymes known as trypsins produced in the pancreas.

The Krebs had discovered a natural, drugless method to help prevent cancer. But their discovery wasn't original. Years prior to any of the Drs. Krebs' works, Drs. George B. Wood and Franklin Bache, MD, published a reference volume in 1833 in which they described amygdalin, derived from B17, as a common treatment for a wide range of diseases and disorders.

Vitamin B17 is also referred to as a nitriloside, which is the foundation for Laetrile, amygdalin, and prunasin. Together with the pancreatic enzyme trypsin, these can form a natural barrier against cancer growth. If foods containing any of the nitrilosides are eaten regularly, the body's own immune mechanisms can naturally battle cancer-forming cells. But if foods containing these critical vitamins are not regularly consumed (or manufactured), nature's mechanisms can't work as effectively against the buildup of factors at the root of cancer and the countless number of degenerative diseases.

This is happening to human beings today. Not only are advanced societies environmentally polluted to dangerous levels, but also more and more foods are being altered from their natural state by man's own doing. Modern freeze-dried, fat-free, sugar-free, calorie-free, weight-watchful, microwavable artificial food substitutes don't contain nitrilosides. *Most food manufacturers don't even know what nitrilosides are.* Never in human history have artificial foods saturated with preservatives and unhealthy chemicals dominated the food supply to the degree they do today. Modern nourishment is no longer nourishing.

In the late 1970s, Dr. Harold W. Manner, PhD, Chairman of the Biology Department at Loyola University, Chicago, Illinois, studied the overall value of Laetrile (B17). His work was well respected and considered among the first unbiased studies since the Krebs' in the 1920s. He reported Laetrile as being virtually non-toxic.

When Dr. Manner used Laetrile in his medical research, along with vitamin A and digestive enzymes, he discovered the production of antibodies was stimulated against spontaneous breast tumors in his laboratory mice. He studied the results of complete regression in 76% of the treated mice with mammary gland cancers. Dr. Manner believed Laetrile received its best results when used in conjunction with digestive enzymes, a traditional balanced diet, and with vitamin A. (This is one of the principles of good ayurvedic or herbal formulations.)

No physician has had more clinical experience with Laetrile than Ernesto Contreras, Sr., MD, of the Contreras Hospital in Tijuana, Mexico, formerly The Oasis of Hope Hospital. Dr. Contreras has clinically used Laetrile for more than forty years on thousands of terminally diagnosed patients and has received impressive results.

One of Dr. Contreras' patients was a man suffering from severe colon cancer. Using Laetrile treatments in conjunction with detoxification protocols and proper vitamin supplementation, Contreras was able to arrest the progression of his patient's cancer. The man lived more than fifteen years beyond his predicted death.

The following is a list of foods rich in vitamin B17:

- Watercress
- Spinach
- Bamboo sprouts
- Alfalfa sprouts
- Lentil sprouts
- Whole nuts
- Mung bean sprouts
- Ground nuts
- Garbanzo sprouts
- Apple seeds
- Apricot seeds
- Strawberries

The basic fact that must be understood with regard to the prevention of cancers and in preventive medicine is that drugs do not prevent diseases from developing but on the contrary can initiate and accelerate the development of disease conditions due to their toxicities, as a result of which we see their side effects in patients. Some of these side effects arise from the excess free radicals that are generated from the metabolism of these chemicals while others can arise from their destructive effect through oxidative stress on biomolecules in the tissues in which they target, including adhesion molecules that can lead to internal bleeding as the integrity of the cementing material that binds cells together is destroyed over time. Chemo-drugs, like aspirin and other anti-inflammatory drugs have such capacity.

The answers to preventive medicine are found in nutrition from a broad range of antioxidants obtained in the bioavailable form from food and edible substances. Bioavailable means the mineral or phytochemical is available for immediate and direct use in the body's biochemistry. Minerals from organic sources are bioavailable such as the minerals found in fruit juices and inside the egg but the calcium in the eggshell is not bioavailable, although it is in a food source because it is bound in ways that is not easily broken down and released in the free form for use in the body's biochemical reactions and its consumption does not, for instance, reverse osteoporosis. Nutrition from food and edible sources is an integral part of healthy biochemistry and it supports such healthy biochemistry. Hence, clinical nutrition has important application in therapy including in slowing down the progress of disease states. Nutrition is not just about the quantitative methods and approaches that ensure that a person gets enough of water, protein, fats and carbohydrates but rather has a special focus on dietary intake of bioavailable minerals from organic sources, a broad range of antioxidants and fat-soluble antioxidants and medium chain fatty acids. It is an important issue in patients and for maintaining health. Inorganic minerals are not advised for patients as these are not water-soluble and not bioavailable. Plants can uptake inorganic minerals from the soil and convert them into the organic forms that are then used to build the phytochemicals and natural L-form antioxidants.

Vegetables, fruits, and whole grains contain a wide variety of phytochemicals that have the potential to modulate cancer development. They also have phytochemicals that can form conjugates that help to transport macromolecules such as glucose across membranes. There are many biologically plausible reasons why consumption of plant foods might slow or prevent the appearance of cancer. One of the key reasons is that with sufficient antioxidants through food sources, the oxygen free radical is quickly converted into water and oxygen by the body's natural antioxidant system. This system requires organic minerals for its enhanced catalytic function. This process, when it is efficient, eliminates the potential for oxidative stress. Hence the risk for the formation of secondary radicals (e.g. the hydroxyl radical) and the highly reactive peroxynitrite oxidant is not present. The hydroxyl and the peroxynitrite oxidant and other secondary radicals can cause harmful and detrimental damage to free molecules and molecules bound in cell membranes by robbing electrons from them. The useful molecular function of such oxidatively-damaged molecules is lost and they may then participate in forming harmful free radical chain reactions. Oxidatively-damaged cell walls lead to chronic inflammation and the development of disease conditions such as psoriasis, arthritis, cancers etc while oxidative damage to mitochondrial membranes invariably leads to the mitochondrial origin of disease states such as cancers and fatigue and tiredness as the biochemical pathways leading to the formation of ATP are disrupted or when the Krebs cycle is suppressed. Drugs and chemicals like pesticides can suppress the Krebs cycle in the mitochondria. However, cancer patients should not take herbs rich in glutathione, as this enzyme is used by cancer cells to protect the toxic iron-sulfide chemical pathway in them which produces other toxic chemicals that promote the development of the cancer cells into bioreactors that in turn enables the growth of tumors. Phytochemicals that help to disrupt or shut down this iron-sulfide chemistry in cancer cells can help to shrink tumors as opposed to the use of substances like apricots, which in proper administration together other antioxidants can effectively promote apoptosis in cancer cells in a manner that is biologically selective.

Fruits and vegetables and spices also have phytochemicals that are anti-inflammatory which work in synergy with the antioxidants that nature has packed in them. Hence, turmeric, garlic, cloves, black pepper and ginger have anticancer properties as reported in recent studies that do not use distillates as heat destroys the molecules and the natural antioxidants. Potential anticarcinogenic substances in fruits and vegetables include carotenoids, chlorophyll, flavonoids, indole, isothiocyanate, polyphenolic compounds, protease inhibitors, sulfides, and terpenes. The specific mechanisms of action of most phytochem-icals in cancer prevention are not yet clear but appear to be varied. Considering the large number and variety of dietary phytochemicals, their interactive effects on cancer risks may be extremely difficult to assess. Phytochemicals can inhibit carcino-genesis by inhibiting phase I enzymes, and induction of phase II enzymes, scavenging DNA reactive agents, suppressing the abnormal proliferation of early, preneoplastic lesions, and inhibiting certain properties of the cancer cell.

All of these foods are useful in prevention and in clinical nutrition, but their potential declines when the person or patient has protozoal infection as well, simply because these protozoa feed on vitamin B12 at night and secrete allergens that are very toxic and can set up chronic inflammations leading to the devel-opment of disease states including cancers, skin conditions and arthritis. Protozoal infections are much more common than is currently recognized. At least 25% of the American population is suffering from vitamin B deficiencies. Your doctor will not tell the underlying cause of such a deficiency, its relation to possible protozoal infections and the association of protozoal infections and oxidative stress marked by a decline in blood antioxidant levels in cancer patients. The role of oxidative stress in the initiation of disease states is now clearly understood and recognized and the reversal of disease states in patients with oxidative states depends very much on natural antioxidant and minerals from organic sources. There is the need to understand the role of protozoa in health and disease and to also consume food and edible herbs with anti-parasitic properties.

## Chapter 3

# Of self and others

*Another popular myth of Pulp Med is that of a self-contained and self-confined organism. Interactions of micro and macro environments are usually ignored. Pulp Med, being a selfish medicine itself, treats organisms as selfish and isolated. This is again a catastrophic approach that excludes a huge array of interactions that play a vital role in health and sickness*

*We have to understand that each and every one of us is an ecosystem. A large part of our DNA is made of viruses, mitochondria probably originated from the symbiosis of two species, microorganisms constitute our intestinal flora and produce for us biochemical products essential for our survival and well-being. It is all about balance, equilibrium. The notion of the "Other", of the non-self as a constant threat will turn out to be Catastrophic.*

### a) Why doctors will give you only half truths about...
**Mitochondria, Self, Health and the Universe**

One fundamental characteristic of the current civilization is selfishness permeating all levels and spheres of human existence: from the individual perceptions of being, to the social implications of co-existing, to the economic theories of managing and turning co-existence into a profitable network, to the environmental issues of ecologic co-dependence and to the scientific innovations that promote knowledge in all of the aforementioned fields and in even more, selfishness has governed and spawned most of the theories and practices that we today encounter. This solipsism, this egomania, this perception that only I and Mine exist and are worth serving, saving and caring for has already created huge financial problems with the 2008 crash, and is creating even huger environmental problems that no one can confidently predict if and how we are going to be able to resolve and restore balance to our cosmos. In other words, this approach, though a sometimes admirable driving force of the Western world, has an innate limitation: it considers expansion of "self" and exploitation of others as limitless. But since space exploration is underdeveloped, for the next decades we are bound to live in a "sphere" called earth, a world whose limits are well defined and known, a limited world not a limitless one. When expansion has reached exhaustion, when new sources, ideas, innovations, markets, technological breakthroughs are hard to find, when "self" has expanded to such a degree that it can no longer transpose or transfer or dump its problems into new grounds, into fresh "others", once self has become almost "everything", at least everything it knows and owns of the cosmos, than "self" has to encounter all of the problems of the "others" that it has by now conquered, phagocytosed, incorporated. And when this time comes, "self" is left only two options (actually only one but for the sake of argument we'll propose that there are two). One is to try to survive by metamorphosing, to become more introvert, reinvest some of the dynamics of the expansionistic aggressiveness onto solving the internal problems by creating more detailed and extensive networks and regulations and attempt to stabilize and redefine this uncontrollable "self". This is a model of internal expansion, of expansion within one's self, an introspective approach. The other is to attempt to expand further at the same or higher rate than previously when expansion is no longer viable and to ultimately collapse, collapse onto itself like a black hole.

There are many paradigms that attest to the nature and outcome of expansion in a limited world. It begins with marvelous aggression, almost unobstructed, until it reaches its limits. Historically, all universal empires collapsed from within, when they could no longer sustain expansion. Rome lasted longer because it transformed some of its aggression into administration. In cosmology, if expansion speed does not overcome the escape velocity, the world will contract (and finally collapse), possibly back into a universal pre-Big Bang state. In biology, a cell culture grows geometrically until the nutrient substrate is exhausted. Then the culture starves to death and diminishes (in a sense collapses onto itself) until the proper ratio of available nutrients is restored. In the sociologic and financial Malthusian model, overpopulation can exhaust the planet's available resources and lead to war, famine or both, again in a sense collapsing onto itself (off course Malthus took into consideration only overpopulation and not – as he should have done – also overexploitation).

That is what universally happens when expansion is no longer sustainable but it is still perceived as indefinite: collapse.

The sense of self and infinite expansion onto others has these implications in all other aspects of human activity and thought. But what about medicine?

Medicine and biology in general is fraught with selfish perceptions. From the Darwinian survival of the fittest to the neo-Darwinian selfish gene, from antidrugs (antibacterial, antiviral, anticancer etc.) to a genetically governed world, all these disciplines teach us of is Self. Self is good and must be preserved, non-self must be destroyed or controlled. Even cancer, which is a bizarre immortal yet often lethal and ultimately self-destructive expression of self, is treated by medicine as a non-self, as the enemy that has to be destroyed. Since the human body is limited and well defined, expansionism is expressed in exerting control and destroying the others. But even this introvert by nature expansion of self has limitations. Because – as the immune system knows all too well – the notion of self in medicine cannot be taken literally.

Our own genome consists also of incorporated inert (most of the time) viral genetic material. Our own intestinal flora consists of non-self bacteria, vital for our survival and well-being. And our own cells contain cell organelles that billions of years ago were non-self and still are not completely subjected to our cellular government of the nucleus.

We call them mitochondria. They are our power plants. They are matriarchally inherited to us. They have their own DNA (mtDNA) which is independent from our "core" DNA, the biological essence of our being and fate as "macho" medicine wants us to believe. They are not just organelles that are centrally and absolutely governed by core DNA. They are essentially symbiotes, merged with our viscera in our cellular ancestors billions of years ago, giving us now the energy we depend upon in order to live.[78]

When needed they multiply to provide our tissues with additional energy. But their DNA is also more sensitive than core DNA. They don't have the complexity and the longitude of the core DNA repair system. So they get damaged more easily. And when they get damaged or depleted they can lead to or get involved in any type of non-infectious disease states one can imagine. Imagine a factory without power or with a shortage of power. It can be completely dysfunctional or the administration can choose to shut down sectors to save power for the most important ones. Some or all workers in the factory will work in the dark. Occupational accidents will happen. If there is a general power shortage, the factory, no matter what the administration decides to do, will dysfunction or ultimately shut down. Our civilization will be seriously impaired or shut down if faced with serious energy shortages. There is no need to argue that our body will definitely do the same, deteriorate or die.

There are few to thousands of mitochondria in each cell. Each mitochondrion in turn contains multiple copies of mtDNA. This variable mitochondrial numerology has many implications and complications for health and for disease expression, duration, extent and severity. As it has been accurately described in the proceedings of the June 2008 NIH's National Institute of Neurological Disorders and Stroke June 2008 workshop on Mitochondrial Encephalopathies and potential relationship to Autism:

> "...mutations in mtDNA may affect all copies of mtDNA (homoplasmy), but frequently they only affect some copies (heteroplasmy). Since the many copies of mtDNA are distributed randomly between daughter cells during cell division, heteroplasmy can lead to significant variation in the proportion of mutated mtDNA over time and across different organs or tissues. This variation in mutation load can influence the clinical expression of mitochondrial disease. Heteroplasmy may also complicate the diagnosis of mtDNA diseases because the causative mutation may be present in only some tissues, such as specific brain regions or specific muscles, and not in others, such as blood or hair. In addition, an individual's mtDNA haplotype can modify the effect of pathogenic mutations in mitochondrial genes. More broadly, mtDNA haplotypes may also modify susceptibility for diseases in which mitochondrial dysfunction may not be a primary cause, including diabetes, multiple sclerosis, and some cancers and neurodegenerative diseases."[79]

One has to understand the complexity and the diversity of mitochondrial involvement in health and disease states. Mitochondrial deficiency, damage, inefficiency, mutation or any combination of the previous mitochondrial states does not manifest itself homogeneously, and may effect certain cells or tissues of the body or be systemic or even catholic. It may be sudden or slow or cataclysmic or acute or chronic or degenerative, episodic, chronic or both, triggered or remain "dormant", with mild or severe symptoms or no symptoms at all or with subclinical symptoms that may not be necessarily associated to a disease state, such as fatigue and restlessness. It might contribute to other disease states or be affected by other disease states. It might even be associated with dysmotility, migraine, depression,[80] anxiety,[81] mood or other psychiatric disorders.[82] In depression and especially in depression with somatization low energy production and mitochondrial dysfunction has also been indicated.[83] The reverse process, that is whether depression with somatization causes mitochondrial dysfunction which in turn aggravates depression, should be also examined as this loop is in accordance with the "positive feedback" depression, low self-esteem and reduced motivation and physical mobility progression. And it is not only about non-infectious diseases. Infectious diseases can also cause direct damage to mitochondria complicating things even further.[84] And there has been a novel discovery indicating that mitochondria play also a vital role in immune response and thus that mitochondria are vital in fighting off infections and especially RNA-Viral infections such as flu, hepatitis, West Nile Virus, SARS (and possibly the so-called HIV infection). A protein named MAVS (Mitochondrial Anti-Viral Signaling protein) located in mitochondrial membrane plays an initial role in triggering immune response against viruses:

> The researchers modified normal cells so that the cells could not produce the MAVS protein, which is short for Mitochondrial Anti-Viral Signaling protein. Without MAVS, the cells were highly vulnerable to infection with two common viruses in a class called RNA viruses  Other RNA viruses include hepatitis C, West Nile, SARS and the flu viruses.
>
> Cells altered to produce an overabundance of MAVS were protected from dying from viral infection.[85]

On the other hand, one of the key elements of the biochemical chain of events that comprise an immune response (co-triggered, as suggested, by MAVS) is interferon. Interferon has the ability to inhibit mitochondrial DNA expression and therefore function. As research suggests: "We showed previously that type I interferon causes a down-regulation of mitochondrial gene expression. We show here that IFN treatment leads to functional impairment of mitochondria...

Possibly as a consequence of the inhibitory effect on mitochondrial gene expression, treatment with interferon causes a reduction in cellular ATP levels. The inhibition of cellular growth by interferon may thus be partly a consequence of a reduction in cellular ATP levels."[86] Furthermore there has been some mitochondrial involvement indicated in autoimmune diseases.[87]

So, in this long chain of events and counter-events, of effects and counter-effects, it is very hard to distinguish cause from effect, first from second. The mitochondrial realm is not governed by some linear strictly-deterministic rational, but it rather works in circular patterns with intertwining positive and negative feedback mechanisms. It is not about intervention, it is about balance. It is not about attacking or prohibiting. It is about regulating, coordinating and tuning. It is not only about finding and defining. It is about understanding, understanding the big picture. And these are tasks that the overspecialized lab-rat scientist will fail to address over and over again, tasks that Big Pharma will either ignore or conceal.

One has to completely understand that any kind of non-infectious, infectious, immune, autoimmune, acute, chronic health conditions, large or small, direct or indirect, primary or secondary may present mitochondrial involvement.

Let us examine some more aspects of the mitochondrial realm. For reasons of achieving better understanding biochemical events are more often than not described as linear and organelles and cells are described as if static. The universally-accepted truth is that most systems are not static. They are dynamic. The cell world is fluid, it is a sea. Shape shifting and motility occur over time and that is also the case with mitochondria. The questions of shape and motility play a vital role in biological events and have not been properly addressed so far. Mitochondria are mobile elements[88] in a mobile world. The mitochondria do not eternally retain a morphological integrity. They also fuse with each other, exchanging components and materials,[89] in a cellular ritual that one could describe as "mitochondrial sex". This is the actual world of mitochondria, a mobile world and a dynamic environment, not a textbook schematic or even an electron microscope picture. It is poetry in motion. And poetry is very hard to be understood by stagnant lab-rat scientists who don't understand or feel or write poetry.

Mitochondria are pivotal, critical, beautiful. They are life givers, life providers. One could say that mitochondria are life. And as expected, as in all things living, they are also death.

Mitochondria are associated with cell apoptosis. Mitochondrial damage is not only associated with disease but also with aging and, ultimately, death. There can possibly be some events of cataclysmic mitochondrial damage and some inherent mitochondrial diseases that can make a kid have the mobility and energy of elders, but usually, due to the complexity of the mitochondrial system, damage caused by drugs, toxins, age, malnutrition are accumulating over time before they reach a threshold and start to produce evident or measurable health effects.

Let us examine some of the things that can possibly make our mitochondria and us sick, old and ultimately dead.

Free radicals: drugs, pesticides, smoking, chemicals, environmental toxins can ultimately damage our mitochondria. Most of the free radical-inducing substances are explored in other chapters of this book. In this point we are going to examine some of them that are not:

As mitochondrial DNA is more susceptible to damage, it has been suggested that chemotherapy and radiotherapy can cause point mutation of mtDNA. As a relevant research indicates: "Our studies have shown that in patients who have been treated for cancer there is an increased level of mtDNA damage."[90]

Methotrexate, a potent chemotherapeutic and antirheumatic agent, exhausts folic acid and subsequently purines, inhibiting DNA and of course mtDNA synthesis, leading progressively to mitochondrial depletion

Another agent under investigation for the treatment of cancer in combination with chemotherapy is buthionine sulfoximine, a synthetic amino acid that inhibits gamma-glutamylcysteine synthetase, thereby depleting cells of glutathione. Glutathione is a metabolite that plays a critical role in protecting cells against oxidative stress in free radical-induced apoptosis. Through extensive depletion of glutathione, buthionine sulfoximine damages muscle cell mitochondria and leads to skeletal muscle degeneration. The damage can possibly be prevented by co-administration of glutathione monoester.[91]

And mitochondrial damage does not only involve chemotherapeutics, or rather it doesn't involve only cancer chemotherapeutics. Another class of chemotherapeutics that block essential cellular functions, the AIDS chemotherapeutics and especially RTIs (Reverse Transcriptase Inhibitors) cause mitochondrial depletion or damage. The dreaded and disfiguring lipoatrophy is only one, perhaps the most obvious RTIs side effect on mitochondria.[92] There are possibly many, many, many more RTIs related mitochondrial damage consequences that are there to be explored and addressed. This is a possible side effect drug profile that was from the very beginning obvious to anyone who had the capacity to think straight. RTIs inhibit reverse transcriptase. Mitochondria employ reverse transcriptase. Thus, RTIs would logically damage mitochondria. Yet, despite that obvious reason, relatively little research was done on RTI and mitochondrial damage in relation to research done on RTIs therapeutic benefits. Why is that?

What about other "virus specific" antiviral treatments? Ribavirin used for example in hepatitis C treatment, in combination with RTIs, works synergistically in inducing increased mitochondrial toxicity.[93]

But it is not only antiretrovirals that damage mitochondrial DNA. Let us not forget that mitochondria are of bacterial origin so antibiotics seem perfectly able to undo them. And they do undo them.

Antibiotics called aminoglycosides, used to treat chronic bacterial infections such as tuberculosis, may attack mitochondria on people that specifically have an MT-RNR1 gene mutation and cause deafness. This is of course a somewhat rare but very real adverse drug reaction.

Another class of antibiotics, sulpha compounds like cotrimoxazole (Bactrim, Septrim), used until recently also in acne treatment, block the synthesis of tetrahydrofolic acid, the metabolically active form of folic acid and subsequently the synthesis of purines,[94] arresting mitochondria from producing DNA and gradually depleting them. Heavy metals can do the same.

Other antibiotic classes like fluoroquinolones, macrolides, clindamycin, rifampin, tetracycline, and especially chloramphenicol and linezolid have been also shown to impair mitochondrial function.[95]

Valproate, an anticonvulsant and mood stabilizer can damage mitochondria and some statins can also do this. Natural neurotoxins, some fungal toxins and chemicals such as MPTP and the insecticide rotenone can also damage them.

Now imagine this: an AIDS patient taking RTIs for AIDS, radiotherapy for persistent KS (Kaposi's sarcoma), chemotherapy and radiotherapy for non Hodgkin's lymphoma and different classes of antibiotics for opportunistic infections.

All of the above cause mitochondrial damage through different biochemical pathways. Or imagine any other combination of the huge array of mitochondrial killers in a body. This is biochemical havoc, a mitochondrial genocide. Now add to this free radical and toxic accumulation and what do get? A dead or at best a chronically-impaired patient. Even if anyone was to survive the underlying medical conditions, none can survive for long without mitochondria.

In the beginning of the previous century, an eminent biochemist and Nobel laureate Otto Warburg made an elegant hypothesis. He proposed that cancer derives when cells shut down their aerobic respiration and turn anaerobic and that in a sense the cell and mitochondria symbiosis is dissolved (Warburg phenomenon), a forced divorce. Heinrich Kremer revitalized the theory and expanded it also in AIDS to face fierce critique and persecutions.

It is obvious, in our fragile little cell quests, the mitochondria are absolutely essential and are involved in an incalculable number of disease and health conditions that have been ignored by research. Even conventional medicine can understand this. As mentioned in the 2008 workshop:

> Though much is known about some specific mitochondrial diseases, our understanding of how mitochondrial function and dysfunction contribute to the broader scope of human disease is incomplete and evolving, and the workshop panelists emphasized a growing recognition of the many ways that mitochondrial function can be disrupted. They suggested that mitochondrial disease may be more common than currently thought and will likely be implicated in an increasing number of medical conditions, including aging and cancer.[96]

There have been some treatments proposed to avoid or limit or repair or reverse mitochondrial damage, to avoid or limit disease conditions and to promote well-being and perhaps longevity. The use of antioxidants seems rational since free radicals damage mitochondria as well. There should be no arguing over this. Free radicals cause damage, antioxidants scavenge them. The real issue is an issue that occupies conventional medicine and should also occupy alternative disciplines of medicine: how to deliver substances to where they are essentially needed. The issue of antioxidants and supplementation should be an issue not of pharmacology in general but rather an issue of pharmacokinetics.

Bruce Ames, an eminent molecular biologist and the inventor of the Ames test, has been studying the process of aging for years; he actually grew old studying the state of oldness. There are few that have studied mitochondrial involvement in aging as well as Ames. And he is still at it. He supplemented rats with a combination of two common dietary supplements, acetyl-L-carnitine, an acetylated form of L-carnitine that transports fatty acids from the cytosol to mitochondria where they are metabolized for the production of energy, and alpha-lipoic acid, a known antioxidant. The results were impressive as Ames narrated: "With the two supplements together, these old rats got up and did the Macarena. The brain looks better, they are full of energy, everything we looked at looks more like a young animal," he said.

"We did two different tests for cognitive activity in rats, and in both it made a big difference to feed them this mixture. Memory degenerates with age, and this makes them better."[97] Two other nutrients, vitamin B1 (thiamine) and/or B2 (riboflavin) are required cofactors for the conversion of adenosine diphosphate (ADP) into the "bioenergy currency" adenosine triphosphate (ATP) have been suggested to be mitochondrial friendly. Furthermore, they have been suggested to repair certain types of mitochondrial damage. According to research:

Nucleoside analogue-induced lactic acidosis is an often fatal condition in patients with HIV. There is only one report of successful treatment with riboflavin. We describe a 30-year-old female with AIDS and nucleoside analogue-induced lactic acidosis that exacerbated shortly after introducing total parenteral nutrition and reversed within hours after the addition of thiamine. Successful treatment of nucleoside analogue-induced lactic acidosis with a high dose of thiamine supports the hypothesis that vitamin deficiency is an important cofactor in the development of this rare and unpredictable condition in patients with HIV. We suggest that high dose B-vitamins should be given to any patient presenting with lactic acidosis under nucleoside analogue treatment.[98]

Antioxidant vitamin E and ATP recharger co-enzyme Q-10 might also have applications to prevent mitochondrial damage and promote mitochondrial function.

We have referred to expansion vs. exhaustion models and suggested that they are universal. Health clearly expands to the point where mitochondria (energy) are exhausted. After this point it collapses. The suggestions of mitochondrial supplementation are just rough drafts of a future medical science that will promote energetic living instead of pathetic being, will adopt a dynamic interpretation of cellular life instead of a static one. There is so much we don't know about mitochondria, cell symbiosis and balance that we can only dare to make suggestions on how to treat them and implications of how their abuse is deteriorating or jeopardizing the future of the health of our generation and the future of the health of coming generations. The royal cellular theory of a nucleus-governed organism with histones as the royal courtyards, RNA and proteins as merchants and everything else as laypeople has expanded to the point of exhaustion. The steady, stable, well arranged and totalitarian universe, governed by law, god, a principle, DNA, kings, priests, tycoons and specialists has expanded so much that it has already reached exhaustion. It is time for new dynamic models to reappear in all fields and especially in the most stagnant of them, Medicine.

A quantum like revolution in biology has to come about soon. And we have to better understand and accept the meaning of the word equilibrium: both sides of the scale in balance.

*b) Why doctors will give you only half truths about...*
**Viruses and Vaccines**
The word 'virus' comes from the Latin for a poisonous liquid, and before that from the Sanskrit for the same. The hunt for them started when, towards the end of the 19th century, it was suggested that invisible living particles much smaller than bacteria might cause the epidemic illnesses for which no bacterial cause could be found. When the electron microscope found tiny particles in the blood serum of patients entering and leaving human cells, this was a Eureka Moment. The prediction was surely about to be proved true. These particles were assumed to be invading and hijacking our cells in order to reproduce. They were thus all condemned as poisons, as 'viruses'.

As more of these were searched for and found in sick people, many illnesses became blamed on them. They became the invisible enemy, the nano-terrorist we must fear. We were instructed that one of our first duties for our newborn children is to vaccinate them against this dreaded foe. Thus was created an ever-growing multibillion-dollar pharmaceutical industry.

But, as I have traveled through the science that underlies this industry, I have gradually learned to ask questions. I now realize that there is another way to see this story that fits all the data. I have learnt from biologists that our cells naturally produce viral-like particles without being invaded or infected, both when healthy and sick. Currently such particles are named by asking what illnesses they cause as if this is their raison d'être, their only importance, the sole reason for cells making them. They would be named far more positively and comprehensively by asking what cells produce them and for what purpose.

Scientists like Barbara McClintock, who won a Nobel Prize for finding that cells operate with intelligence and seek to repair themselves, have given us a very different understanding of the particles they make. We now know that our cells create multitudes of tiny transport particles (vesicles) to carry the proteins and genetic codes needed within and between cells. The ones that travel between cells – those our cells use to communicate with each other – are puzzlingly just like those that we have long blamed for illnesses.

It now seems that we may have broadly misconceived the virus; that they may be simply inert messages in envelopes carried from cell to cell. In the last ten years scientists have begun to call them instead 'exosomes', particles that leave the body of the cell, thus removing the inference that they are all poisons. Distinguishing the healthy particle from the pathogenic is now an enormous problem for the virologist, for it has been discovered that our cells make them all in the same way, in the very same place. It also seems we cannot stop this process without risking severely damaging our cells.

So, perhaps we need to halt the juggernaut of virology with its virus hunt, and look to see if there is another way of helping us keep healthy. We need to know how we can strengthen the malnourished cell, rather than use the many medicines that try to prevent it from making particles by interfering with its essential processes. We need to know if a poisoned cell may produce unhealthy messengers or viruses. We need to learn far more about cells – for only now are we starting to understand how they communicate and the very important role played in this by the particles we had totally demonized as viruses.

I spent over 4 years in the 1990s researching why the vaccines made to protect our children from viruses sometimes instead did them grievous damage. It then took me over 8 years to travel from accepting without question that a virus causes polio and another causes AIDS to discover that most people, including myself, have been vastly misled.

I now realize that science today is so specialized that every new generation of scientists has had to trust that those who laid the foundations got things right, for they cannot repeat this earlier work except at great cost. If this trust ever proves to be misplaced it is absolutely vital to correct this with all speed and courage.

I have been horrified to learn from the highest scientific authorities that this trust has sometimes been very grievously misplaced. For example, high-level US governmental inquiries in the 1990s, guided by eminent scientists, explicitly reported the key foundation HIV research papers were riddled with grave errors and deceptively "fixed". But when the Republican Party gained control over the US House of Representatives at the end of 1994, it ended this most important investigation, buried its reports and left the scientific papers it found to be erroneous uncorrected. These same papers are thus still frequently used by unsuspecting scientists worldwide, who cite them as proof that HIV causes AIDS.

When I dug back further, to the origins of virology and the great hunt for the poliovirus, I found the story was scandalously much the same. Powerful evidence was presented to Congress linking the summer polio epidemics to summer-used heavy metal pesticides. These scientists suggested remedies, reported curing polio and were ignored. Instead parents were told to be scared of a yet undiscovered virus. Today thousands of children are still being identically paralyzed in regions where such pesticides are heavily used – but all the World Health Organization says is: "Don't worry; we have nearly exterminated the dreaded poliovirus. We have checked. The paralyzed children were not infected by it."

As for childhood vaccinations, surely they have proved a great benefit? I long thought so, but I have found the government scientists we entrust with our children's lives have admitted, at official vaccine safety meetings, that they cannot clean these vaccines; that they allowed their use despite knowing that they are scandalously polluted with numerous viruses, viral and genetic code fragments, possibly toxins, prions and oncogenes. The World Health Organization has also disclosed at these meetings that it has long known the MMR vaccine to be contaminated with avian leucosis virus. This is a bird virus linked to leukemia, but the public have not been told about this. Why most children are not falling ill from this dangerous contamination is, it seems, because most are thankfully gifted by nature with very effective immune systems – and because these viruses are generally not as dangerous as these scientists believe.

As for the great flu epidemic of 1918, it is used today to spread fear of viruses. Yet, shortly after it occurred, an eminent Yale University professor reported that bacteria primarily caused it, and the flu viruses present were virtually harmless. As far as I can discover, his work remains unquestioned but not mentioned. As for the recent scare over bird flu – any self-respecting bird would fall ill and create new viruses if subjected to the amounts of pollution now emitted in China. What we need to focus on is the pollution – not to waste a fortune on chasing genetic code fragments in birds healthily migrating thousands of miles.

What also of the many eminent scientists who have concluded publicly that the HIV theory of AIDS must be scientifically flawed because their research indicates that it has other causes and is curable? Is it right that their research is being suppressed, ridiculed and not funded – simply because they have not confirmed the establishment's theory for this dreaded epidemic?

When I began some twelve years ago my journey into medical research, it took me into the grim world of the virus hunters, a world of selective science and harsh politics.

Highly Contaminated Vaccines

I met with the top government regulatory scientists at the NIH Emergency Workshop on SV40 in 1997. A year later they met again in Washington for another workshop on vaccine safety. At this there were representatives of all the major US government health organizations and of the vaccine manufacturers. A third similar meeting would be held a year later in 1999.

The main issue at the November 1998 meeting was whether or not it would be safe for manufacturers to produce the viruses needed for vaccines from cancer cells. Pharmaceutical companies were at that time seeking government approval for this, on the basis that cancerous cells, as 'immortal' and permanent, would be cheaper to use than cells they had to regularly replace by, for example, buying more monkeys.

These workshops looked at the issue broadly by comparing the safety of the different ways available for making our vaccines. As everyone present was a scientist, the discussions were much more open and frank than they are when journalists are present.

They started with the Measles, Mumps and Rubella vaccine (MMR). One of the first speakers on this was Arifa Khan from the federal Food and Drugs Administration, and what she had to report was very disturbing.

'Today I would like to present an update on the reverse transcriptase activity that is present in chicken cell derived vaccines.' My attention was immediately grabbed. I knew that the mumps and measles viruses used for the MMR vaccine are grown in fertilized chicken eggs, as are also the viruses for the Flu and Yellow Fever vaccines. (The rubella virus for MMR is produced differently – in artificially-grown cells taken originally from an aborted human fetus.)

Dr. Khan was reporting the result of a just concluded two-year investigation into the safety of MMR led by the World Health Organization. She explained that this was initiated in 1996 after the discovery in MMR of Reverse Transcriptase, an enzyme whose presence they believed could well indicate that retroviruses had contaminated the vaccine. This had greatly alarmed them as some retroviruses are thought to cause cancers – and AIDS.

WHO had then quietly, without telling the public, without withdrawing the vaccine, organized MMR safety studies at various laboratories to see "whether this reverse transcriptase activity was associated with a retroviral particle, and even more importantly, whether this retrovirus particle could infect and replicate in human cells."

What they then discovered confirmed their worst fears. Dr. Khan continued: "The reverse transcriptase activity is found to be associated with retroviral particles of two distinct avian endogenous retroviral families designated as EAV (Endogenous Avian Virus) and ALV (Avian Leukosis Virus). Now ALV stands for Avian Leukosis Virus. It is associated with a leukemia cancer found in wild birds, so definitely was not wanted in the vaccines. EAV was, however, less dangerous, at least for birds, as it is natural for them to have it."

Dr. Khan added that they had also found another possible danger: "There was a theoretical possibility that the virus [ALV "Avian Leukosis Virus" ] could ... infect the [human] cell" thus integrating its genetic code into the human DNA to cause cancer. The only reassurance she could give was that her team had watched vaccine cultures for a full "48 hours", and, in that time period, no merger of viral and human DNA had been observed. I thought this was much too short a period to guarantee safety. Cancers develop over years.

Dr. Khan then warned: "There is a possibility that there could also be potential pseudotypes (merging between)... the measles vaccine virus and the retroviral sequences" – meaning there was a risk that bird viruses might combine with the measles virus in the vaccine to create dangerous new mutant viruses. They had not seen it, but it could happen.

She acknowledged much longer term safety studies were needed than 48 hours, but said that long-term studies of measles vaccine cultures were very difficult: "because the measles vaccine virus itself lyses [kills] the culture in about three to four days." This had prevented them from studying the longer-term consequences of this contamination of the MMR vaccine.

So far, she added, they had only managed to analyze a small part of the retrovirus contamination in the vaccines. "Our ongoing studies are directed towards doing similar analyses of other retroviral genetic codes found in the vaccine preparations." It was suspected that other retroviruses might also be present. She also noted that "about 20 years ago similar reverse transcriptase activity was reported" in the vaccine. Apparently nothing had been done about it at that time and the public were never told.

She concluded by explaining what the World Health Organization had decided to do about this chicken leucosis virus contamination.  It would take the risk of quietly allowing MMR to continue to be contaminated. It would permit vaccine manufacturers to continue to use retrovirus contaminated eggs, because "you cannot get ALV free flocks in places where you are making yellow fever vaccine."

Dr. Andrew Lewis, head of the DNA Virus Laboratory in the Division of Viral Products, then warned: "All the egg-based vaccines are contaminated," including "influenza, yellow fever and smallpox vaccines, as well as the vaccine for horses against encephalomyelitis virus" for "these fertilized chicken eggs are susceptible to a wide variety of viruses."

This was an eye opener for me. Before I started on this investigation, if I thought about it, I would have presumed our vaccines were made of selected viruses in sterile fluid to which a small amount of preservative chemicals has been added. I think this is what most parents presume.

It was thus a shock to discover from this top-level scientific workshop that the viruses in our current vaccines are not in a sterile fluid as I had presumed, but in a soup of unknown bits and pieces, a veritable witches' brew of DNA fragments, added chemicals, proteins and even possibly prions and oncogenes, all of which would easily pass through the filters used to be injected into our children.

Our vaccines, I thus learned, are not filtered clean but are suspensions from the manufacturers' 'incubation tanks' in which the viruses are produced from 'substrates' of mashed bird embryo, minced monkey kidneys or cloned human cells. These suspensions are filtered before use but only to remove particles larger than viruses. The point of the vaccine is that it contains viruses, thus these must not be filtered out. This means there remains in the vaccine everything of the same size or smaller, including what the manufacturers call 'degradation products' – parts of decayed viruses or cells.

I also learned that the only official checks made for contaminants in vaccines are for a few known pathogens, thus ignoring a vast host of unknown, unstudied small particles and chemicals. These eminent doctors reported at these vaccine safety meetings that it is simply impossible to remove these from our common vaccines – and this would of course also apply to vaccines for pets, farm animals and birds.

I went to the published reports of the MMR manufacturers and found these confirmed what the scientists at this workshop had reported. A manufacturer stated in 2000 that it made the MMR vaccine with 'harvested virus fluids'. It stated frankly, that their "Measles vaccine bulk is an unpurified product whose potency was measured through a biological assay for the active substance rather than through evaluation of integrity of physical form. Degradation products are neither identified nor quantified." In other words, it left the latter in the measles vaccine along with all contaminants that lay there quietly, or worked slowly. The pharmaceutical company admitted checking the measles vaccine only for obviously active contaminates. It did not measure how much the vaccine was polluted with genetic code fragments, other viruses, or with parts of bacterial, animal, bird or human cells.

The latest information I could find on the retroviral contamination of the MMR vaccine was in a 2001 scientific paper from the CDC (Centers for Disease Control). This reported that 100 MMR recipients were tested to see if they were contaminated by either of the two types of retroviruses identified by Dr. Khan and others. The conclusion was dramatic. "The finding of RT (reverse transcriptase) activity in all measles vaccine lots from different manufacturers tested suggests that this occurrence is not sporadic and that vaccine recipients may be universally exposed to these [chicken] retroviral particles."

They then concluded: "Despite these reassuring data, the presence of avian retroviral particles in chick embryo fibroblast-derived vaccines [like MMR ] raises questions about the suitability of primary chicken cell substrates, the cells used for virus-producing cultures for vaccine production." They recommended considering stopping production in fertilized eggs, and growing the vaccine viruses instead on "RT-negative cells from different species, such as on immortalized [cancerous] or diploid [laboratory grown] mammalian cells." I was amazed to learn this, for, to the best of my knowledge, nothing has been done since this report was made to render MMR safer. The measles vaccine is still produced from contaminated chicken embryos.

All ways of making vaccines have their dangers. Dr. Hayflick, a well-reputed scientist involved for many years with vaccines, described how the 'Primary Culture' method of taking cells from 'sacrificed animals' or bird embryos ran into problems when "*it became apparent that these cells contained many unwanted viruses, some of which were lethal to humans."* He noted: "Latent viruses were such a problem with primary monkey kidney cells that a worldwide moratorium on the licensing of all polio virus vaccines was called in 1967 because of death and illnesses that occurred in monkey kidney workers and vaccine manufacturing facilities." The contaminating virus then blamed was the deadly Ebola. This was most serious, but again I could find no record of the public being informed about this suspension or the Ebola.

The top UK government expert present at this conference, Dr. Phil Minor, of the National Institute of Biological Standards and Control, added that the polio vaccine had originally been so polluted that its doses contained as much monkey virus as poliovirus! I had no idea that so much monkey virus was in this vaccine given to hundreds of millions of children. Then there was another shock for me. I had been assured two years earlier at the SV40 (Simian Virus 40) Workshop that the poliovaccine was no longer contaminated with SV40 – and consequently I had so assured the UK public in our resulting Channel 4 television documentary. Now I learned I had been misled and consequently had seriously misinformed the public. Scientists reported to this meeting that 'SV40 sequences' remained in the poliovirus seed used for the current polio vaccines.

Dr. Heyrick told of how the eminent Dr. Maurice Hilleman had used what he thought was an 'intestine-based cell line' to make an adenovirus vaccine, only to discover to his horror that his cell line had been invaded and taken over by the aggressive cervical cancer virus known as HeLa.

I also learnt that DNA fragments contaminating vaccine lots might be from dead cells but nevertheless remained extremely active and dangerous. Dr. Golding feared they might combine with other genetic codes contaminating the vaccine lots – and thus create a mutant viral strain that could even get in the individual doses of vaccine.

The removal of this contaminating DNA has proved impossible. The US government in 1986 recommended a weight limit for contaminating DNA of 100 picograms per vaccine dose. But the manufacturers could not meet this safety recommendation, as was explained at this workshop. Their failure again led the government to relax its standards, applying the 100 picograms limit solely to vaccines produced from cancerous cells, and allowing one hundred times as much contaminating DNA (10 nanograms) in vaccines produced on other types of cells. But the meeting was told that vaccine manufacturers now admitted they could not meet even this lower standard of 'purity'. Thus high levels of hazardous DNA pollution remain in many vaccines.

This failure was a great concern to the meeting. Many of the doctors present worried that such a great amount of DNA fragments might cause viral mutations in the vaccines. 'Naked' DNA (with no protein coat) is known to be highly reactive. Dr. Phil Krause calculated:

If there are 10 nanograms of residual DNA per dose, which is the current WHO recommendation, and if two doses were recommended per child, as is the case with MMR vaccine, and the infectivity of viral DNA in the vaccine were comparable to that of purified polyoma virus DNA, we can calculate the theoretical infectivity risk. ... For a vaccine that is universally administered to the 4 million children born in the US every year, this would represent about 500 infections per year, clearly an unacceptable rate.

This shocked me. If he was right, and it seemed he was (none of the experts present questioned his calculations), this surely meant the current MMR vaccine is potentially very dangerous. Krause also had only added up the risk from the one vaccine. What when to it is added the contaminating DNA in all the other vaccines?

Dr. Krause also stated: "Of course, in the context of DNA vaccines, we are talking about injecting even larger quantities of DNA into people." He was speaking here about the new DNA vaccines being developed as 'safer' than our current vaccines.

Another important safety issue was raised. "What would this contaminating DNA do when it was injected into humans in vaccines? Could it change our own DNA? Could it cause cancers – or autoimmune diseases?" "When you consider that almost every one of these vaccines is injected right into the tissue that is the preferred site for DNA gene therapy ... I think you couldn't do much more to get the DNA expressed [to get contaminating DNA taken up by human cells] than to inject it into a muscle in the way it's being done." Another speaker lamely admitted: "I chaired the committee that licensed the chickenpox vaccine, and it [residual DNA] was actually an issue that we considered at that time. We looked among recipients of the vaccine for evidence of an autoimmune response associated with the DNA included in that vaccine." He then added: "Actually, we didn't look, we asked the company to look and they did not find one."

Walid Heneine of the CDC asked: "No one has mentioned how much DNA we now have in the licensed vaccines. I mean, how much are we being exposed to? Do we have any idea how much is in the viral vaccines, like yellow fever, measles, mumps vaccines? Do the regulators have an idea from the manufacturers how much DNA there is?"

Dr. Loewer replied: "I have no idea. Nobody that I know has mentioned it." Dr. Becky Sheets from CBER then confirmed the suspicions of many when she responded: "I think that the vast majority of licensed vaccines, US licensed vaccines, have not been tested for residual DNA. The few that have been tested are the ones that have been licensed in the last few years, including varicella and hepatitis A."

She then added: "I wanted to respond to an earlier question regarding how purified are live viral vaccines [like MMR] – [the answer is] minimally purified."

These presentations made some of the experts very uneasy. Dr. Desrosiers stated: "I don't worry so much about the agents that one can test for. I worry about the agents that you can't test for, that you don't know about." Dr. Greenberg agreed. He said he was: "worried also about the agents that aren't known." He continued: "There are still countless thousands of undiscovered viruses, proteins, and similar particles. We have only identified a very small part of the microbial world – and we can only test for those we have identified. Thus the vaccine cultures could contain many unknown particles." Another doctor said: "As time goes on, of course, new viruses are discovered and new problems arise. The foamy virus has been [recently] identified as one that we should be really sure is absent from these vaccines."

The chairman of the workshop then asked Dr. Maxine Linial: "Maxine, does anybody know if vaccines have been checked for foamy virus contamination?"

She replied: "As far as I know, no."

"You mean nobody has looked or as far as you know?"

She responded: "I don't know. There are very few reagents. I mean, there are reagents for the so-called human or chimp foamy virus, but as far as I know, there are no good antibody reagents." In other words, they could not tell if the vaccines contained foamy viruses. ('Reagents' are antibodies to known virus particles.)

The experts voiced other concerns. "And I'll be honest and say that I'm surprised that primary African green monkey kidney cells continue to be used, and I'm a little bit disappointed that FDA and whoever is involved had not had a more serious effort to move away from primary African green monkey kidneys. We all know that there are a number of neurodegenerative conditions and other conditions where viral causes have been suspected for years and no viral agent identified. Maybe they're caused by viruses, but maybe they're not."

Another doctor said: "We need to consider again some of the issues of residual DNA. Is it oncogenic? We had a lot of experience with chicken leucosis viruses in chick embryo cells beginning back in 1960. And the thing about them is they are not easy to detect because they don't produce any pathogenic effect."

An unnamed participant added: "I have to express some bewilderment [at this talk of dangerous contamination], simply because, as I mentioned last night, the vero cell, which under many conditions is neoplastic [cancerous], has been licensed for the production of IPV and OPV [the common polio vaccines] in the United States, Thailand, Belgium and France." The current polio vaccines thus run the risk of having oncogenes in them. Again this was news to me. I had no idea that the polio vaccine might be grown on cancer cells.

Dr. Rosenberg added, unreassuringly: "When one uses neoplastic cells as substrates for vaccine development, one can inadvertently get virus to virus, or virus to cellular particle, interactions that could have unknown biological consequences."

Dr. Tom Broker said we had to be concerned about "papillomavirus infections" in the vaccine... "One of the more remarkable facts of this family of diseases is that since 1980 more people have died of HPV disease than have died of AIDS."

Dr. Phil Minor told of another disaster. "Hepatitis B was transmitted by yellow fever vaccine back in the 1940s. The hepatitis B actually came from the stabilizers of the albumin that was actually put in there to keep it stable."

He continued: "For many years, rabies vaccines were produced in mouse brain or sheep brain. They have quite serious consequences, but not necessarily associated with adventitial agents. You can get encephalitis as a result of immune responses to the non-invasic protein." "Influenza is an actuated vaccine. Again, it's not made on SPF eggs, that is, specified pathogen-free eggs. They are avian leukosis virus free, but they are not free of all the other pathogens that you would choose to exclude from the measles vaccine production system."

Dr. Minor, the UK's top vaccine safety officer, then added: "So even today then you have to bear in mind that a large amount of vaccine that's made is made on really quite crude materials, from an adventitious agent point of view. It's not a trivial usage. In fact, when you consider what vaccines are actually made on these days, they are quite primitive in some respects."

These warnings were coming from a doctor working for the UK government who asked me at a later meeting not to pass on vaccine information that would alarm parents.

He went on to discuss SV40 and the polio vaccine. "It's a very common polyoma virus of old world monkeys, and particularly rhesus macaques. The difficulty with this was that, when the rhesus macaque monkeys are sacrificed and a primary monkey kidney culture made from him or her, as the case may be, a silent infection is set up. So there is evidence of infection [found] just by looking at the cultures. In fact, these cultures can throw out as much SV40 as they do polio [virus]." "The problem was that the cell cultures didn't show any sign of having defects, when they were actually infected with SV40."

It seemed that SV40, and its accompanying proteins and genetic codes, would never have got into so many humans if they had not contaminated the vaccine – and that they were only dangerous when moved into a species for which their presence was not natural – such as into humans and into cynomolgus (African Green) monkeys.

Dr. Minor continued: 'Wild caught monkeys were being used extensively in vaccine production. Up to a half of the cultures would have been thrown away because of adventitious agent contamination, mainly foamy virus, but certainly other things as well."

But, they could not be certain what viruses were present. They could be mistaking SV40 for other viruses. Why? He explained because antibody tests are used to test for its presence

– and such tests are not all that accurate. Antibodies don't only react to a specific viral protein. They may 'cross-react' against other things. "What you could also argue is that you are not picking up SV40 specific antibodies at all, and they could be other human polyomas [viruses] like the BK or the JC, and it's cross-reacting antibodies that we're picking up. I think that is still a thing that needs to be resolved."

"The point about this long story which I have just been telling you about SV40 is that SV40 was a problem between 1955 and 1962, and it's now 1999, and we still don't really know what was going on. So if you actually make a mistake, it's really quite serious. It may keep you occupied for the rest of your working life.'

Then Dr. Minor made a still more alarming admission: "Now the regulatory authorities in the room will be well aware of a large number of other examples of this type which don't actually get published. I think that's not so good. I think this stuff really should be out there in the public literature."

Another UK expert then took the stand. It was Dr. Robertson from NIBSC and, as he explained, "For those of you who don't know, NIBSC is CBER's cousin from across the pond in the UK." In other words, it was the top UK vaccine safety monitoring body. He started off on a reassuring note: "There is no evidence for any increase in the incidence of childhood cancers since the onset of measles, mumps vaccination." But he then said: "But, I think, as a scientific community, unless we do something at least for the future, we might be in a very difficult situation to defend certain issues. If I confronted some of the violent ideologically pure Greens in our country, [telling them what we have been discussing here] I'm sure they would say, 'Shut it down because this is unsafe, totally unsafe.'"

It was thus that I learned that our vaccines are a veritable soup, made up not just of viruses that should or should not be there, but also thousands of bits of viruses and of cells, DNA and

RNA genetic codes, proteins, enzymes, chemicals and perhaps oncogenes and prions. The vaccine was monitored for the presence of only a very few of these particles and vaccine lots are thrown away only if these are found.

*A Vaccine Link to Autism?*

I have not mentioned one final addition to the vaccines – the preserving and antibiotic chemicals added to the doses. The manufacturer of a MMR vaccine noted: "The finished product contains the following excipients: sucrose, hydrolyzed gelatin (porcine), sorbitol, monosodium glutamate, sodium phosphate, sodium bicarbonate, potassium phosphate and Medium 199 with Hanks' Salts, Minimum Essential Medium Eagle (MEM), neomycin, phenol red, hydrochloric acid and sodium hydroxide." What these chemicals might do was not discussed at these workshops.

On top of this I knew from government records that vaccines sometimes contain the pork-derived trypsin used to break up monkey cells and other flesh in the vaccine cultures. Also, in the latest version of the Salk vaccine there is a surprisingly large amount of formaldehyde left behind after it has done its work of 'poisoning the viruses' (despite biology teaching us that viruses are not living particles). These workshops omitted all these from their consideration.

Today the Salk vaccine is back in use under the brand name IPOL, supposedly in a safer format – and the Sabin is now out of use in the West as it is now blamed for causing some polio cases. But IPOL officially "contains maximum 0.02% of formaldehyde per dose." This is 200 parts a million, yet a major Harvard University study on the CDC website reports: "Formaldehyde is a reactive chemical that has been recognized as a human carcinogen. At levels above 0.1 parts per million, the exposure causes a burning sensation in the eyes, nose and throat; nausea; coughing; chest tightness; wheezing; and skin rashes."

This utterly shocked me. It added to the horror of these workshop reports which show our top government scientists report that our children are vaccinated with 'primitive' cocktails of viruses among DNA fragments, chemicals and cellular debris, all potentially highly dangerous – along with many unidentified particles.

Furthermore a transcript of an Institute of Medicine June 2000 meeting of scientists from the CDC, FDA and vaccine industry reveals it was called because a CDC scientist, Dr. Thomas Verstraeten, found a statistically significant relationship between mercury in vaccines and several neurological conditions, including possibly autism, which today is seriously affecting many of our children.

The official US Environmental Protection Agency safety of exposure standard for mercury is 0.1 microgram per kilogram of body weight per day, or 7 micrograms for a 70-kilogram adult. Yet, "fully vaccinated children receive as much as 237.5 micrograms of mercury from vaccines in doses of up to 25 micrograms each." According to 2003 research, "thimerosal [mercury] in a single vaccine greatly exceeds the EPA adult standard."

And yet, undeniably, most of our children seem to survive multiple doses with these vaccines with no evident damage. How can this be?

My horror at discovering how little is known about the contents of our vaccines is counterbalanced by my growing admiration for our marvelous immune system. Apparently after vaccination, if we are in a good state of health, it normally is quite capable of neutralizing much of this debris, removing or reducing its great danger.

But this did not explain why top scientists, who believe with every iota of their being in the great danger presented by viruses, who see these as the great enemy, have exposed our children to such dangers, without ever informing the public of these risks?

In 2002 further research found major childhood vaccines

contaminated with retroviruses. "The reverse transcriptase-positive vaccines include measles, mumps, and yellow fever vaccines produced by several manufacturers in Europe and the United States. RT activity was detected in the vaccines despite strict manufacturing practices requiring that chick embryos and embryo fibroblasts be derived from closed, specific pathogen-free chicken flocks. Such chickens are screened for known pathogens."

The authors also stated: "Endogenous retroviral particles are not addressed by current manufacturing guidelines because these particles had not been associated with chick cell-derived vaccines." But this is not so. Their paper admits: "The presence of Avian Leukosis virus (ALV) in chick cell-derived vaccines is not a new phenomenon; many instances of ALV contamination in yellow fever and measles vaccines have been documented." As far as I am concerned, the "current manufacturing guidelines" should have been adjusted to take account of this.

The research paper continued: "The finding of reverse transcriptase activity in all measles vaccine lots from different manufacturers tested suggests that this occurrence is not sporadic and that vaccine recipients may be universally exposed to these retroviral particles."

So far, however, they had not detected these chicken retroviruses in the children vaccinated. But their results so far were inconclusive, they admitted. "Confirmation of our molecular results by EAV-specific serologic testing may however be necessary. The lack of evidence of transmission of EAV [Endogenous Avian Virus] to vaccinees is likely due to the presence of defective particles. No infectious EAVs have yet been isolated, nor has a full-length intact EAV provirus been identified. However, our understanding of the EAV family is limited."

Their final conclusion: "Despite these reassuring data, the presence of avian retroviral particles in chick embryo fibroblast-derived vaccines raises questions about the suitability of primary chicken cell substrates for vaccine production..."

They suggest the measles and other egg-grown vaccines should be grown instead on "immortalized or diploid mammalian cells" but added a caveat: "Since the cell substrate is critical to the attenuation of live vaccine viruses, any change in the cell substrate could have unpredictable effects on the safety and efficacy of the vaccine and should be approached cautiously."

It thus seems that the reason why so far little has been done to remove the chicken virus contamination from the MMR and other vaccines – is that there is no known safer way to vaccinate, despite many decades of research, and the governments spending millions of dollars to try to find a safe way to make vaccines. Toxins accumulate in the body – so what long-term cumulative damage is being caused through the great numbers of vaccines given today?

Measles, mumps and other vaccines continue to be produced on contaminated fertilized bird eggs. WHO and the national health authorities have quietly, but officially, permitted childhood vaccines to contain 'a low level' of viral contamination – simply because they cannot remove it economically.

WHO currently approves as acceptable a level of contamination of 106 to 107 possible viral particles per milliliter for the substrates on which our vaccines are grown. They publicly say this only presents a "theoretical safety concern" but clearly they still wonder, as they did at the conference, if they are right and if it might be safer to grow the vaccine viruses on cancer cells.

Vaccines have become very big business since more and more doses per child are stipulated and purchased every year. The estimated revenue from childhood vaccines in the US is now over 2.4 billion dollars a year. But is the contamination in the vaccines now producing many sick children?

Today there are reports from parents and doctors of increasing numbers of children falling ill after vaccination and developing Autism. It is reported that this may be due to damage to their cells' mitochondria from the toxins accumulating from vaccines. Three-quarters of the autistic children tested in one study had damaged mitochondria.

A CDC report had claimed to prove that vaccines could not possibly be causing autism. Both the US and UK governments had cited this in defense of the vaccine program. But the CDC has since been forced to admit to Congress that this report was flawed and inaccurate. It turned out that the first time they processed their statistics for this report these revealed a significant risk that vaccines had caused these illnesses – but then the authors had removed a quarter of the susceptible cases and this, with other unjustified recalculations, reversed the results.

This was unearthed only after "in 2005, a group of Senators and Representatives headed by Sen. Joe Lieberman wrote to the NIEHS (an agency of the National Institutes of Health) saying that many parents no longer trusted the CDC to conduct independent-minded studies of its own vaccine program. Lieberman et al asked NIEHS to review the CDC's work on the vaccine database and report back with critiques and suggestions." The NIEHS had come back with a severely critical report.

In 2007 it was accepted by a US court, and by government experts, that vaccination played a significant role in making autistic the nine-year-old child Hannah Poling. This major test case opened the door for compensation for many in a fast-growing autism epidemic. The US government at first tried to play down the significance of this by saying Hannah's disease was mostly due to her having a small DNA mutation in her mitochondria – but her mother has the same and has never fallen ill. Hannah also did not fall ill – until June 20, 2000, when she had 9 vaccines on the same day. It was also accepted by the government that the fits she suffered were a result of these vaccinations, although it took 6 years of illness before they began. It seems the damage done by vaccination can take years to unfold.

On February 21, 2008, the US government made a second concession. In court documents it agreed that Hannah's 'autistic' brain disease was 'caused' by vaccine-induced fever and overstimulation of her immune system. She may have had slight damage to her mitochondria from environmental toxins but she had no symptoms of illness – prior to these 9 vaccines.

Mercury might prepare the ground for autism along with other vaccine pollutants, pesticides and environmental hazards. They might damage the mitochondria, but it is the cumulative effect of vaccination that seems to finally overwhelm the child's health, for many parents report their child's illness began within hours or days of a vaccination that was not the first given to the child. This is not surprising. Toxins accumulate in the body. They may do no harm at first – but when they reach a critical level, then they can overwhelm the child's health. The evidence produced shows that there is far more pollution in children's vaccines than has been widely known of until now. It is criminal that our public health authorities have kept silent about this until now.

Some autistic children have been reportedly treated with some success by having their blood detoxified and with regular oxygen-breathing sessions – thus removing some of the toxic contaminants and assisting the damaged mitochondria – but even this has not led, as far as I know, to a full recovery.

I should mention here a consequence of having too many vaccine jabs in the same arm muscle. This can cause paralysis in that arm, a disorder known clinically as 'provocation polio'. This surely is clear evidence of the damage that can be done by the accumulation of vaccine toxins?

Then of course there are the cases of epilepsy in children following MMR that started me on this investigation, particularly the brain-damaged child of the courageous John and Jackie Fletcher.

Nevertheless, doctors responsible for public health continue to reassure us on television that our vaccines are proved totally safe and effective, while behind closed doors, and in court, it is now clear that these same experts are saying something else entirely. In private they acknowledge our current vaccines are based on primitive science and have many worrying risk factors. Even the replacement vaccines on the horizon, spun to us as safer, are not proving safe in the laboratory. Up until now, parental concerns have mostly been about the additives put in the vaccines – such as mercury and aluminum salts – but this evidence suggests that the very nature of the vaccine manufacturing process provides the major dangers.

In other words, the vaccines we give our children are liquids filled with chemicals and a host of unknown particles, most of which came from the cells of non-humans: from chickens, monkeys, or even from cancer cells. Truly we do not know what we are doing or what the long-term consequences are. All that is known for sure is that vaccines are a very cheap form of public medicine often provided by governments to ensure the public that they really do care for the safety of our children.

*c) Why doctors will give you only half-truths about...*
## The Aliens Within
"Most conventional doctors do not recognize the symptoms of Candida overgrowth, and are clueless about how to cure it."[99] There are similar problems with protozoal infections, especial in detection and when the symptoms are subclinical.

Psoriatic skin conditions are often lumped together as psoriasis but blood investigations may show fungus or heavy metals or protozoal infection as the underlying cause other than a block in Coenzyme Q10 and natural corticosteroid in the body (or suppression by excess medicant-drug use) and these conditions must therefore be treated accordingly but there is little hope from the allophatic pharmacy for fungal psoriasis or due to heavy metal free radical chain reactions or protozoal infections that cause the chronic inflammations or to detox the body of inorganic minerals in supplements or medicant-drugs that tend to bioaccumulate in fat cells of the body. Many disease states and degenerative disease conditions arise from chronic inflammations in which the cell membrane integrity is affected to the extent that it alters cell output and cell function. Chronic inflammations occur when natural antioxidant levels are low and are caused by:

1. Excess free radicals, including the superoxide and secondary free radicals such as the hydroxyl and the peroxynitrite oxidant,
2. Heavy metals that can initiate free radical chain reactions,
3. Afflatoxins produced by fungal infections,
4. Viral toxins such CMV virus toxins or hepatitis B virus toxins, and
5. Protozoal allergens.

Protozoal infections go undetected simply because, upon infection, the molecules that compose their cell structures and their excretions and secretions are allergenic to the tissues and the body responds by encapsulation to "cordon them off" but over the long term their allergens can cause havoc leading to arthritis, persistent cough that gets worse at night, skin rashes that develop into bad dermatitis with increased itch at night, corn formations, chronic hypertension that gives a high reading in the morning and tends to lower towards the evening, a high blood sugar reading (FBS) that tends to lower towards the evening, eyesight and ocular problems as well.

The encapsulation response of the body explains why protozoa are not easily detected through blood tests. They are held in these tissue capsules. One tablespoon of turmeric formulated with other edible herbs mixed with a cup of warm water and taken orally like a tea about 4 minutes later appears to flush out the protozoa. A blood test done about 20-22 minutes after consumption shows the parasites in the blood, if there was an earlier infection. We have observed protozoal infections in cancer patients as well and these are usually "heavy". Smokers who develop cancers tend to have heavy metals as well as protozoal infections. Micro-nodules in lungs may be indicative of protozoal infection.

Protozoa are not symbiotic in nature, unlike symbiotic bacteria that flourish in the large intestines. They feed on the best of nutrition including vitamin B12. They become active at night. Their feeding activity at night and consequent secretions and excretions at night are increased that lead to increased inflammatory activity at night. Hence, there is greater intensity of itch in skin rashes and greater irritation in the throat at night in patients with persistent cough. Vitamin B12, a natural antioxidant, is found in nerves and neuropathy of nerves can set in, even in the patient whose blood sugar levels are well within normal limits. Vitamin B12 is important in the regulatory processes including in hormone production, the amount of LDL production in the liver and a chronic protozoal infection of the liver can result in raised LDL levels at night. The depletion of vitamin B12 and the increased inflammatory activity caused by the protozoal allergens explain the "Dawn Phenomenon" or Somogyi Effect, in which not only blood sugar levels become raised but LDL may also be raised at dawn. Protozoal allergens are disruptive to the formation of the GTF factor that is critical in glucose passage and entry into cells and it can have an oxidative effect on hormones including insulin directly. LDL molecules may also suffer similar oxidative injury thereby increasing the risk of plague formation, lowering of libido and possibly prostrate problems. A large percentage of fertility problems may also be attributable to protozoal infections, especially if these are lodged in the lining of the womb. Another problem associated with eye problems and problems related to vision may be directly attributable to protozoa in the ocular tissue.

Treatment with B vitamins or food rich in niacin such as wheat grass, for patients in certain conditions such as skin rashes or persistent cough that gets worse at night or for neuropathies, can have counter results as it only serves to feed the protozoa. Naturally taking extra insulin at night for patients with Somogyi is not a viable long-term solution as it would deplete more natural antioxidants in the body and slowly create more complications.

Protozoa-induced chronic infection may also be responsible for many of the degenerative kidney conditions and chronic hypertension and problems in the lining of the womb that can prevent implantation of the fertilized ovum. All of these need to be further investigated systematically for the advancement of medicine and developing therapies that are non-toxic. Of special interest is to investigate the association of protozoal infections with the incidence of diabetes and breast cancer.

Most parasitic infections are chronic, and the host immune response reacts to the different stages of the parasite life cycle involving different parasite antigens. The chronicity of these infections is characterized by fluctuations in antigenemia and therefore in host responses. Glomerular lesions associated with parasitic infections are observed that lead to the proliferation of glomerular disease through chronic inflammation caused by their allergens. "The association of parasitic infections with glomerular injury is clear. The glomerular lesions observed in parasitic infections cover the whole range of glomerular lesions known, but most of them are proliferative."[100] The host natural immunity comprising parasite antigens appears weak and such weakness is primarily due to the oxidative damage suffered by these antigens by the allergens produced by the parasites that results in chronic inflammation that aids the proliferation of disease.

There is a range of clinical manifestations in glomerulopathy. Different clinical syndromes are associated with each type of glomerulopathy. The clinical manifestations range from isolated proteinuria or hematuria to nephrotic syndrome (proteinuria of >3.5 g/day, hypoalbuminemia, generalized edema, and hyperlipidemia), nephritic syndrome (glomerular hematuria, recognized by erythrocyte casts in the urine, and diminished glomerular filtration with some degree of azotemia, oliguria, and hypertension), renal insufficiency, and rapidly progressive glomerulonephritis (nephritic syndrome with doubling of the creatinine level in serum within 3 months as a sign of progressive renal failure).

Chronic inflammation caused by protozoal allergens can suppress the human immune system and may have a troubling relationship with the spread of AIDS that is not yet properly recognized. Leishmania is a protozoal parasite transmitted to humans through sand fly bites. The allergens may be the primary cause of the destruction of the mucous membranes of the nose, mouth and throat and surrounding tissues, or visceral, resulting in wasting while concurrent infections result in pneumonia and diarrheal disease and bleeding secondary to thrombocytopenia and impaired liver function. In visceral leishmaniasis, the parasite infects macrophages throughout the reticuloendothelial system, compromising the immune system. Malnourished people have relatively lower levels of B vitamins (including B12) and have decreased immunity. Protozoal infections suppress the immune system and accelerate the onset of opportunistic infections (e.g. pneumonia, tuberculosis) and their allergens promote chronic inflammations that aid the proliferation of disease conditions. In malnourished people, as in poor communities in Africa, most patients will be expected to die before their CD4 counts reach the low levels generally observed in seropositive AIDS patients in richer societies as in European communities.[101]

When CD4+ T-cells are fewer than 200 CD4+ T-cells per micro-liter (μL) of blood, cellular immunity is lost, leading to the condition known as AIDS. Protozoal infection of macrophages or the allergenic destruction of macrophages by protozoal allergens can also reduce CD4 cell counts. In a European study, 79–90% of people with HIV-visceral leishmaniasis co-infection were found to have CD4 cell counts of less than 200 106/L.[102] In Ethiopia, most patients die before reaching such low CD4 counts.[103]

Most of the antibiotics that are effective against bacteria are not active against protozoa. Most of the drugs used in the treatment of diseases caused by protozoa are synthetic or from plants. Drugs like metronidazole produce breakages in DNA or suppress DNA replication and are toxic to host cells, too. Quinacrine, used in the treatment of giardiasis, adheres to DNA molecules and results in yellow staining of skin or deposit blue and black pigment in nail beds. Nifurtimox is used in the treatment of flagellated protozoa. Its metabolism yields high amounts of superoxide or oxygen free radicals that are lethal to it and produce oxidative damage to host cells. Most of such drugs are toxic and can produce side effects. Treating glomerulopathy associated with or caused by parasitic infections with drugs that generate large amounts of superoxide to kill parasites can result in further aggravation of the disease through oxidative damage that serves to increase inflammatory damage to cell membranes.

Visceral leishmaniasis (kala-azar) is a worldwide dissemi-nated intracellular protozoal infection for which prolonged, conventional therapy with pentavalent antimony has become increasingly less effective. Relapse may occur in otherwise healthy persons simply because the drug may not pass into the capsule that is encapsulating the protozoa. Relapse also occurs in malnourished people and in people receiving immunosup-pressive therapy.[104] "Most human infections caused by visceral-izing strains of Leishmania are probably subclinical, attesting to innate resistance or, more likely, to T (Th1)-cell-dependent immune responses which induce acquired resistance. While treatment is not given for subclinical infection, remote recrudescence still remains a possibility, especially if the host becomes T-cell deficient.[105] Herein lies the problem in public health coupled with the fact that protozoa stay encapsulated and cannot be seen in live blood analysis but as blood antioxidant levels decline with age, the chronic inflammation caused by their allergens begin to manifest in disease or suppression of the immune system. As T4 cell counts decline, opportunistic infections begin to take root.

A new drug, NTZ (nitazoxanide), the first to be developed in the last thirty years, is now available for treating the three most common causes of protozoal diarrhea caused by Cryptosporidium parvum, Giardia intestinalis and Entamoeba histolytica. The concept of using the fixed combination of trimethoprim and sulfamethoxazole resulted from the recognition that bacteria are obligate folic acid synthesizers, while humans obtain folate through dietary sources. So drugs like trimethoprim and sulfamethoxazole were developed to inhibit bacterial synthesis of tetrahydrofolic acid. Tetrahydrofolic acid is the physiologically active form of folic acid and a necessary cofactor in the synthesis of thymidine, purines and bacterial DNA. However, both drugs cross the placenta and appear in breast milk, with detectable concentrations found in fetal serum in patients undergoing therapy. The problem of killing protozoa that are encapsulated without toxicity to host cells still remains a problem in allophatic medicine and one has to look into research in anti-parasitic phytochemicals.

The proper approach to patients with cancers, arthritis, hypertension and skin conditions is to find a way to flush out the protozoa into the bloodstream. Then a drop of peripheral blood can placed under the microscope for observation. If these are present, then measures must be administered to kill these parasites. In most cases, the symptoms of disease tend to clear up. It also explains why cancer patients with protozoal infections who are in remission from chemotherapy have a high relapse rate. And naturally, all women planning to get pregnant ought to get a protozoal test done before the conception.

Fortunately, there are a number of edible roots and herbs that are antifungal and/or anti-parasitic and have strong anti-protozoal activity that can be used in therapy. However, this therapy has an interesting and inherent complexity. As the protozoa are flushed out from the 'capsules' into the bloodstream they secrete allergens that cause the blood cells to aggregate and appear compacted, about 20 minutes after treatment, in almost the same way that chemo-drugs tightly compact blood cells. That indicates the very high degree of toxicity of allergens produced by protozoa and their ability to induce chronic inflammations that can lead to arthritis, hypertension, CVD, diabetes and cancers. Hence, it is necessary to orally consume a glass of orange and noni juice or use a nano-biotech spray formulated from extracts obtained in the nano-form from garlic, orange, lime and noni. This dermal spray serves as an anti-allergy spray as well and it results in good thinning of the blood within 40 minutes, without disturbance to its clotting abilities, unlike aspirin, depending on the amount sprayed and its concentration. This process can be repeated every day until the condition, such as psoriasis, is resolved and three subsequent blood tests fail to reveal any protozoa.

In hypertensive patients, wherein protozoal infection is a cofactor to problems in nitric oxide biochemistry, the anti-hyper-tensive spray will cause an initial drop in blood pressure followed by a rebound that can be higher than the original depending on the amount of allergens produced by the flushed out protozoa and an anti-allergy spray is necessary to lower the blood pressure.

Protozoal infections can come about by airborne spores and more often through contact with its animal hosts (cats, dogs, goats and cattle). It is submitted that protozoal infections appear to be much more prevalent than commonly thought and is an issue in public health and chronic disease management.

## Chapter 4

# Towards a global health dictatorship

*a) Why doctors will give you only half-truths about...*
**Chemicals and Disease Conditions**
For the environmentally aware, there is no need to describe the
environmental problems we face today. Literally thousands of
books, articles and films have been produced showing that the
biosphere has been dramatically disturbed and chemically
changed by human activities (Ecology 30). But the average
individual may not know that, in 1989 alone, more than
1,000,000,000 pounds of chemicals were released into the ground,
contaminating our farmlands and drinking waters. Over
188,000,000 pounds of chemicals were also discharged into
surface waters such as lakes and rivers. More than 2,400,000,000
pounds of chemicals were pumped into the air we breathe. A
grand total of 5,705,670,380 pounds of chemical pollutants were
released into the environment that we eat, breathe, and live in—
all in just one year (cf: Nicole MR 2002, ISP, College of Lifelong
Learning; Wayne State University). Since WWII, over 80,000
chemicals have been developed and used. Many are pesticides
that degrade soils and contaminate water.

All of these chemicals are toxic to some degree and generate
free radicals that can induce free radical damage in the body.
Some of these chemicals are similar to biomolecules in the body
and they are utilized in metabolic reactions resulting in disease
conditions because their metabolism in the body produces toxic
metabolites or simply because the body cannot differentiate
between them. Their metabolism in the human cells can lead to
excess hydrogen peroxide that must be converted into water and
oxygen by the SOD-catalase-glutathione antioxidant system.

When this process is slow, the excess hydrogen peroxide reacts with the oxygen free radicals (OFR) to yield the highly toxic secondary radical called the hydroxyl radical. The hydroxyl radical is highly reactive and can oxidatively damage cell membranes as well as the genetic molecules. Such damage to the genetic molecules impairs health and can cause developmental defects. A large percentage of pesticides sprayed in gardens, plantations and golf courses end up in the ecology and in ponds and lakes. This explains the significantly large number of frogs with deformities and developmental defects compared to 40–50 years ago.

Free radicals are highly reactive species that can be damaging to the body at the cellular and molecular level, causing oxidative stress to cell membranes, damaging molecules including lipids, hormones and proteins. Those reactive chemicals can damage the cell components and disrupt biochemical pathways by inactivating enzymes involved in the Krebs cycle and receptors for cellular molecules. Since 1985, there is overwhelming scientific evidence demonstrating that free radicals actually contribute to or hasten heart disease, cancer, diabetes, arthritis and other age-related diseases.

Evidence was accumulating over the past three decades that most of the degenerative diseases that afflict humanity have their origin in deleterious free radical reactions. These diseases include atherosclerosis, cancer, inflammatory joint disease, asthma, diabetes, senile dementia and degenerative eye disease.[106]

Since free radicals are involved in carcinogenesis and since some epidemiological studies have suggested that certain antioxidants may reduce cancer risk, some survivors and clinicians might conclude that antioxidants are effective in preventing cancer recurrence[107] while many oncologists believe that antioxidants interfere with chemo-drugs and radiotherapy. The interference is primarily on account of the fact that chemo-drugs and radiation generate large amounts of hydroxyl free radicals that kill cancer cells (as well as normal and healthy cells) and antioxidants scavenge these free radicals. So, while research has shown that free radicals are involved in carcinogenesis, oncologists attempt to treat cancer patients with free radical generating agents as in chemotherapy and radiotherapy.

In fact a study of the relevant literature on cancer risks, whether associated with alcohol, smoking, pollutants, chemicals, toxins or sun exposure (ultraviolet radiation), points to free radicals produced by these agents and/or a poor diet that is low in antioxidants. Put together, it means poor free radical scavenging activity in the body as the primary initiating factor for the risk and the cause of the disease condition and its progress. One way to appreciate the harmful effects of chemicals when introduced into the human body indirectly through the ecology is to understand their effects when they are introduced directly into the human body.

The powerful drugs used in chemotherapy can themselves cause cancer and pose a risk to nurses, pharmacists and others who handle them.[108] Chemotherapy drugs in human and animal studies have shown they have the potential to cause cancer or reproductive problems, said Thomas Connor, a research biologist with the National Institute for Occupational Safety and Health (NIOSH).

Chemo-drugs, like radiation, generate huge amounts of the highly reactive hydroxyl radical that damages cell membranes and disrupts the electron transport system in cells as well as protein synthesis. Natural enzyme and micronutrient levels drop rapidly and that accelerates cell death. Such a new surge of free radicals is generated by chemo-drugs which are cytotoxic to cancer cells as well as normal cells. Thus many young normal cells die due to the treatment. Most of the known carcinogens, including benzene and at least 40 other toxic chemicals in cigarette smoke and pesticides, generate free radicals that create oxidative stress in cells, impairing their aerobic respiration or damaging DNA and mitochondrial DNA, turning them into cancer cells. It is this very same toxicity that is common to carcinogens and chemotherapy-drugs. Hence the NOISH alert really comes as no surprise

Fortunately some of the regulatory bodies are recognizing the dangers of chemicals. The European Chemicals Agency (ECHA) has issued its first recommendation for harmful chemicals that should undergo Europe's new strict 'authorization' process. The EU countries in the ECHA Member States Committee have adopted an opinion supporting the recommendation. ECHA recommend that seven substances of very high concern (SVHC) should be subject to use and market access only with explicit authorization under the EU's REACH law.[109]

Over the last 100 years, sperm count in males is declining while breast cancers in females have been rising. This phenomenon coincides with the increasing use of chemicals in industry and in medical science. Interestingly, three of the seven chemicals proposed by ECHA are officially classified in Europe as toxic to reproduction. One is officially classified as carcinogenic and three are recognized as being persistent, bioaccumulative and toxic (PBT) or very persistent and very bioaccumulative (vPvB). The flame retardant HBCCD has also been identified as a persistent, bioaccumulative and toxic substance by an EU working group, with potential effects on the liver, brain, nervous and hormone systems.

Three chemicals DEHP, DBP and BBP, phthalates or plastic softeners, are already banned in toys and childcare articles in the EU. Medical devices containing DEHP must also be labeled according to the revised European Medical Devices Directive. These phthalates (which become more powerful when present simultaneously), are examined in a recent report on male reproductive health disorders. The existing knowledge about the contribution of phthalates to human testicular disorders points to the need to reduce people's exposure to phthalates, especially pregnant women.[110] Polls show that the public is concerned that the environment may be playing a crucial role in health and disease conditions, and many respondents consider that the EU is not doing enough to address this aspect in prevention, education and policy. The real concern is rooted in the fact that "over the last 50 years, the incidence of cancer has increased rapidly. The officially recognized risk factors for cancer, including age, genetics, smoking, lack of exercise and so on, are unable to account for the rise in incidence for other cancers."[111] This concern is well founded and can be better understood in the way chemicals create problems in the mammalian biological systems.

Wherever there are cells that are rapidly dividing as in the testicles for production of sperm and where there is fatty tissue the relative risk increases sufficiently to result in health concerns and higher risk to the development of disease states. Toxic chemicals tend to interfere with cell division while on the other hand they tend to bioaccumulate in fatty tissue. They can also generate free radicals that rob electrons from hormones leading to problems like diabetes in people with excess visceral fat and breast cancers in women as female breasts have fatty tissue.

Another reason is attributable to the fact that metabolism of chemicals leads to depletion of minerals in the body, especially iron, manganese, zinc and copper. The metabolism of these D-form substances yields a lot of hydrogen peroxide that must be converted into water and oxygen, failing which its reaction with the oxygen free radicals (OFR), the secondary radical called the hydroxyl is formed that is highly reactive and very deleterious to health. These minerals, in the organic and bioavailable form, work in the body's natural antioxidant system to catalytically enhance the role of the natural antioxidant system to convert hydrogen peroxide into water and oxygen.

It is therefore not surprising at all that a report, commissioned by Health and Environment Alliance's (HEAL) partner organization CHEM Trust, titled "Male Reproductive Health Disorders and the Potential Role of Exposure to Environmental Chemicals", written by one of the world's leading experts in reproductive biology, Professor Richard Sharpe of the Medical Research Council (MRC) in Edinburgh, UK, reveals that many everyday chemicals in the environment or in consumer products have the potential to block the action of testosterone, and a baby's exposure to this mixture of chemicals may undermine this process and harm future male reproductive health. Birth defects in male genitals, low sperm counts and testicular cancer, collectively called Testicular Dysgenesis Syndrome (TDS), may all have their origins during development in the womb. The link is convincingly proven in the report as it highlights animal studies that have clearly established that certain hormone disrupting chemicals, in particular testosterone disrupting chemicals, can cause TDS-like disorders.[112]

Bisphenol A (BPA) is employed in the manufacture of a wide range of consumer products. It is an endocrine disruptor that at amounts to which we are exposed alters the reproductive organs of developing rodents has caused concern, if not alarm. At present, no information exists concerning the exposure of human pregnant women and their fetuses to BPA. There is broad human exposure to this chemical.

In a study, blood samples were obtained from healthy premenopausal women, women with early and full-term pregnancy, and umbilical cords at full-term delivery. Ovarian follicular fluids obtained during IVF procedures and amniotic fluids obtained at mid-term and full-term pregnancy were also subject to BPA measurements. The results showed that BPA was present in serum and follicular fluid at 1–2 ng/ml, as well as in fetal serum and full-term amniotic fluid, confirming passage through the placenta. These results suggest accumulation of BPA in early fetuses and significant exposure during the prenatal period, which must be considered in evaluating the potential for human exposure to endocrine-disrupting chemicals.[113]

Regulation is now moving in the direction to ensure that chemicals which act in combination to disrupt hormones are regulated according to their total combined effects (cumulative risk assessment). European Council is likely to adopt the next critical step to establish a definition of "endocrine disrupting" pesticides which will determine which pesticides will be banned.

This is important to properly move towards setting targets to reduce pesticides use and eliminating or restricting pesticides use in public places. Member State targets therefore can and should include significant reductions in the use of hormone-disrupting pesticides; and eliminate their use in public places as soon as possible. However, the problem remains with regard to facilitating their biodegradation upon entering the ecosystems as they can still enter the human body through water and food chains and will come back to create health problems.

Many of the toxic chemicals are used in combination or as a mixture. In mixtures, toxic chemicals will produce cumulative and dose-additive effects.

Scientists have already conducted studies with mixtures to provide a framework for assessing the cumulative effects of "antiandrogenic" chemicals. Rats were dosed during pregnancy with antiandrogens singly or in pairs at dosage levels equivalent to about one half of the ED50 for hypospadias or epididymal agenesis. The pairs include: AR antagonists (vinclozolin plus procymidone), phthalate esters (DBP plus BBP and DEHP plus DBP), a phthalate ester plus an AR antagonist (DBP plus procymidone), and linuron plus BBP. This study proved the expected effects. All binary combinations produced cumulative, dose-additive effects on the androgen-dependent tissues. We also conducted a mixture study combining seven "antiandrogens" together. These chemicals elicit antiandrogenic effects at two different sites in the androgen signaling pathway (i.e. AR antagonist or inhibition of androgen synthesis). In this study, the complex mixture behaved in a dose-additive manner. The results indicate that compounds that act by disparate mechanisms of toxicity display cumulative, dose-additive effects when present in combination.[114]

Chemicals used in pesticides also have antiandrogenic properties and endocrine toxicity. Antiandrogenic chemicals alter sexual differentiation by a variety of mechanisms, and as a consequence, they induce different profiles of effects. For example, in utero treatment with the androgen receptor (AR) antagonist, flutamide, produces ventral prostate agenesis and testicular nondescent, while in contrast, finasteride, an inhibitor of 5-alpha-dihydrotestosterone (DHT) synthesis, rarely, if ever, induces such malformations. In this regard, it was recently proposed that dibutyl phthalate (DBP) alters reproductive development by a different mechanism of action than flutamide or vinclozolin (V), which are AR antagonists, because the male offspring display an unusually high incidence of testicular and epididymal alterations – effects rarely seen after in utero flutamide or V treatment. In one recent study, we present original data describing the reproductive effects of 10 known or suspected antiandrogens, including a Leydig cell toxicant ethane dimethane sulphonate (EDS, 50 mg kg-1 day-1), linuron (L, 100 mg kg-1 day-1), p,p'-DDE (100 mg kg-1 day-1), ketoconazole (12-50 mg kg-1 day-1), procymidone (P, 100 mg kg-1 day-1), chlozolinate (100 mg kg-1 day-1), iprodione (100 mg kg-1 day-1), DBP (500 mg kg-1 day-1), diethylhexyl phthalate (DEHP, 750 mg kg-1 day-1), and polychlorinated biphenyl (PCB) congener no. 169 (single dose of 1.8 mg kg-1). Male offspring display a higher incidence of epididymal and testicular lesions than generally seen with flutamide, P, or V even at high dosage levels. Overall these toxic chemicals display several mechanisms of endocrine toxicity. Ketoconazole did not demasculinize or feminize males but rather displayed anti-hormonal activities, apparently by inhibiting ovarian hormone synthesis, which resulted in delayed delivery and whole litter loss. This study shows the effects of chemicals in pesticides in developmental toxicity.[115]

Bioaccumulation and severe or prolonged exposure to chemicals leads to health problems whose symptoms mimic disease conditions from other causes. When such exposure to chemicals is not understood and taken into account, its treatment is impossible and the patient keeps coming back for more drugs. Unfortunately, conventional treatments are not geared towards the break-up of chemicals in the body and to remove them with non-toxic approaches. Hence, headaches, back pains and symptoms related to or caused by chronic inflammations initiated by free radicals generated by chemicals in the body tend to persist. These health problems can be compounded when there are also populations of protozoa in the body as their allergens also cause chronic inflammation. These protozoa feed on vitamin 12 at night. Symptoms may therefore become more severe at night. In psoriasis patients, the itch increases at night. Such persons may also become deficient in B vitamins especially vitamin B12. Protozoal infections are more common than currently thought and that explains the relatively high incidence of 25% in the US for vitamin B deficiency. Such deficiency in people with protozoal infections can also lead to numbness in hands and neuropathies, chronic hypertension as well as borderline elevations in glucose and LDL levels. Vitamin B12 supplementation only results in a short-lived improvement and the problems can become more aggravated over time as the protozoa feed on the increased supply of vitamin B12 and multiply.

The exposure of people with protozoal infections to chemicals and toxic dust clouds is a problem that needs serious attention and funding for research. The dangers of exposing people and especially pregnant women to hormone-disrupting chemicals in consumer products are now well documented and more members of the public know about it. The focus is on the risks these pose to baby boys and to healthy reproductive biology but compounding factors such as protozoal infections must be also considered. Chemicals can also cause problems in other tissues and organs such as in the dermis and the respiratory tract.

In recent years, cleaning has been identified as an occupational risk because of an increased incidence of reported respiratory effects, such as asthma and asthma-like symptoms among cleaning workers. Due to the lack of systematic occupational hygiene analyses and workplace exposure data, it is not clear which cleaning-related exposures induce or aggravate asthma and other respiratory effects. Currently, there is a need for systematic evaluation of cleaning product ingredients and their exposures in the workplace. Ingredients of concern in cleaning agents include quaternary ammonium compounds, 2-butoxyethanol, and ethanolamines. Cleaning workers are at risk of acute and chronic inhalation exposures to volatile organic compound (VOC) vapors and aerosols generated from product spraying, and dermal exposures mostly through hands.[116] An often overlooked problem with regard to chemicals that affect respiratory health is their impact on the endothelium in the major arteries over time that can lead to disruption in the production of nitric oxide (NO) and the formation of the peroxynitrite oxidant that is also highly reactive species that very often oxidatively damages cell membranes causing joint-pains. Such disruption in the NO yields also leads to hypertension and erectile dysfunction.

Other chemicals found in the environment and in our homes such as formaldehyde can also lead to health problems depending on exposure and period of exposure. Formaldehyde is an economically important chemical, to which more than 2 million US workers are occupationally exposed. Substantially more people are exposed to formaldehyde environmentally, as it is generated by automobile engines, is a component of tobacco smoke and is released from household products, including furniture, particleboard, plywood, and carpeting. The International Agency for Research on Cancer (IARC) recently classified formaldehyde as a human carcinogen that causes nasopharyngeal cancer and also concluded that there is "strong but not sufficient evidence for a causal association between leukemia and occupational exposure to formaldehyde." In a new meta-analysis of these studies, focusing on occupations known to have high formaldehyde exposure, we show that summary relative risks (RRs) were elevated in 15 studies of leukemia (RR=1.54; confidence interval (CI), 1.18-2.00) with the highest relative risks seen in the 6 studies of myeloid leukemia (RR=1.90; 95% CI, 1.31-2.76). The biological plausibility of this observed association lead the researchers to hypothesize that formaldehyde may act on bone marrow directly or, alternatively, may cause leukemia by damaging the hematopoietic stem or early progenitor cells that are located in the circulating blood or nasal passages, which then travel to the bone marrow and become leukemic stem cells.[117] Unfortunately traces of formaldehyde are also found in haze from burning vegetative matter and forest fires.

Although risk assessments are typically conducted on a chemical-by-chemical basis, the 1996 Food Quality Protection Act (FQPA) required the Environmental Protection Agency (EPA) to consider cumulative risk of chemicals that act via a common mechanism of toxicity. The common underlying toxicity of chemicals lies in their ability to generate excess hydrogen peroxide in the body leading to the formation of secondary radicals such as the hydroxyl and the oxidant called the peroxynitrite.

The key issues being the role of chemicals in inducing and accelerating free radical damage and their bioaccumulation in human tissue, it is only proper that we note the interest in exposure assessment that has shifted from pollutant monitoring in air, soil, and water toward personal exposure measurements and biomonitoring. That process is important to assess the level of contamination together with the levels of natural antioxidants in the blood and to monitor both levels against symptoms and health problems. Biochelation procedures and interventions will therefore become the more important and the more critical part of a modern health care system as a large variety of chemicals are already in our environment and more are entering the human body directly through "medications" and indirectly through the ecosystems and through wars that use chemicals to defoliate and weapons that use depleted uranium 235. The lingering health problems of chemical warfare will therefore be astounding if they are surmountable.

The cancer rate in the USA in 1900 was 3 out of 100. Today, 1 in 3 people will get cancer and 1 in 4 will die from it. This amounts to over one million people yearly, killing some 520,000 of us annually. That is one grave problem related to becoming industrialized wherein society is led to use more and more chemicals in industry and at home. In one recent report commissioned by the California EPA done by University of California researchers estimate that in 2004, 200,000 California workers suffered from chronic diseases linked to workplace exposure to industrial chemicals and 4,400 people died of these diseases including cancer, emphysema and Parkinson's disease. New research is beginning to show that low-level synthetic chemical exposure over time can disrupt the natural development of infants and children.

The Collaborative on Health and the Environment (CHE) database report shows links between chemical contaminants and 180 diseases or conditions in humans ranging from skin conditions to fertility to cancers. Chemicals that bioaccumulate in the brain can lead to Alzheimer's and Parkinson's diseases as they cause chronic inflammations in brain cells. The World Health Organization (WHO) has released a report stating that one-quarter of the world's disease burden – and one-third of the disease burden among children – is due to environmental factors that could be modified. Today the human biological system among urban populations is contaminated and so is human breast milk. The chemical origin of diseases must be recognized and included in the medical school program. The problem is paradoxically aggravated by trying to treat symptoms caused by chemicals by other toxic chemicals called drugs that are prescribed as "medications". There is now the need to go for non-toxic treatments and to apply non-toxic pesticides to modify the environment and our ecosystems in order to modify the world's disease burden that is a drag on every economy. In many developed nations it has become a burden on the household.

Business interest sometimes seems to override health concerns. One of the criteria used to lobby in favor of businesses is that the sole basis of hazards based on the toxic properties of a chemical should not prompt its inclusion in Europe's new strict 'authorization' process. But the paradox in medical science still stands which is the use of toxic chemicals to treat health problems. For instance the chemical called AZT which is "toxic by inhalation" and can cause the same symptoms as AIDS is used to treat AIDS patients. Quite naturally, 6 national representatives raised concerns about the inclusion of the flame retardant HBCDD, arguing inclusion on the list could harm small businesses. This goes against REACH which mandates that harmful chemicals be lined up for the authorization procedure solely on the basis of the hazards posed by their toxic properties.

Before toxic chemicals are banned, substance producers or users will have to show that the risks of a particular use can be adequately controlled, or for certain chemicals, that there are overwhelming socioeconomic benefits to the substance's use (that outweigh the health and environment risks) and that no alternatives exist. The real problem is that most of the controls exist only at the production stage and there is little or no control once they are released into the markets and into the ecology.

Health science is beginning to recognize the significance of bioaccumulation of chemicals and chemicals used in pesticides as a cause of persistent pain and chronic disease conditions. Drugs are not a solution to this chemically-induced problem that may be associated with heavy metal bioaccumulation in tissues. The most effective and fast way is to use alpha-lipoic acid and pectins obtained from edible substances in the nano-form to biochelate for safe removal from the human biological system through the urine.

### b) Why doctors will give you only half-truths about...
**The War on Health**
*Can your politician save you from the agenda and designs of Big Pharma? Will your health authorities bother to understand their designs and stand for your health interests?*

I do not think so.

They have too much money to throw around and they have in some cases conspired to create organizations to front for them. They have been very successful in getting more and more toxic chemicals into human bodies in the name of treatment. Some of these chemicals are only marginally more effective than placebos, giving rise to the very good prospect of placebo therapy. No one has bothered to consider this, even though a placebo costs a tiny fraction compared to the drug and it comes with a bonus – no side effects.

Preventive medicine based on nutrition and high antioxidant intake from food sources does not seem to interest anyone except the science-literate consumer because healthy bodies do not contribute to the bottom line of Big Pharma. On the other hand, toxic drugs, once they are legally categorized as medications, can create side effects to be treated by more drugs that positively impact their bottom lines. It is a gravely vicious cycle nurtured through a "cozy" relationship between Big Pharma and the regulatory authorities.

Officials have become so adversarial to ensuring health benefits that they have issued statements to the effect that doctors must only give pharmaceutical benefits to their patients and not health benefits. And, quite naturally, the number of deaths and hospitalizations from adverse drug reactions is increasing every year. But banning toxic drugs for therapy is out of the question. The system has many supporters and these people are in a position to ask for bans on clinical nutrition and to press for those in order to promote their business interests through legislation. Those ridiculous laws and legal definitions will help to stifle the application of nutrition and edible herbs to promote health and for use in therapy unless they are sold by Big Pharma!

*The FDA would also like to harmonize our dietary supplement laws with the evolving international standards set by Codex, thus branding therapeutic nutrition as dangerous and risky and needing to be sold by Big Pharma or removed from the market altogether (if it competes with a blockbuster category of drugs). Codex is planning to use the same proteomics and biomarker technology that will be used by the FDA's Critical Path Initiative to remove therapeutic dietary supplements from the international market and force their policies on America, thereby superseding the sovereignty of American law on threat of trade sanctions. The FDA fully supports draconian Codex guidelines to regulate dietary supplements and is working with the Germans to concoct technology to brand nutrients as drugs.[118]*

The law can define animals as traffic as in the Road Traffic Acts in commonwealth countries. It can be used to distort and warp the natural order of things and a definition can be introduced to even say that vitamin C from fruits is a drug. Where will it all stop? If selling fruits is lucrative, the business can be put in the hands of Big Pharma, by changing the legal definitions. Anything that can be consumed that benefits health, whether it is a supplement or food or anything edible can be redefined in such a way as to make it a business solely of Big Pharma. If it makes money, it can be turned into a monopoly or controlled by changing the legal definitions.

Pharma has embarked on a dirty game because their drugs are not getting any better; they are getting more toxic. And more and more research is showing that these drugs do not work within the natural and healthy biochemistry to provide a health benefit. Hence, the Big Pharma producers are working hard to press for laws and regulations to ensure pharmaceutical benefits instead of health benefits. Let's examine the issue of competition from natural medicine, clinical nutrition, ayurveda and their therapeutic and health benefits that improve quality of life or help to slow down the progression of degenerative conditions. This competition can be killed by legally defining nutrients as drugs so that only pharmaceutical companies can sell them. This becomes all the more critical for them to do as more and more people realize that drugs are D-form chemicals that cause harm in the mammalian L-form biochemistry. Many of these drugs disrupt healthy biochemical pathways by blocking the formation of the ATP molecule or the formation of antioxidant enzymes in the body. They deplete mitochondrial DNA in cells and stores of minerals in the body especially copper, manganese, zinc and iron. Those minerals work catalytically with the glutathione-catalase system to convert hydrogen peroxide produced by the cells' metabolism into water and oxygen, a critical function for maintaining and restoring health. They also deplete magnesium or otherwise suppress your immune system. Some drugs that aim to deliver a pharmaceutical benefit, for example to reduce blood glucose levels by blocking the conversion of lipids into glucose, may end up altering the blood lipid profile, thereby creating a new risk for the patient especially if the patient's antioxidant intake and consumption of soluble fiber through foods is low.

Many drugs generate free radicals in the body. Sometimes these dangers can be easily seen in diabetic patients with diabetic wounds who are given antibiotics resulting in blood sugar levels rising to double the original readings (e.g. from a reading of 7-9 going up to 16-18). On the other hand, Big Pharma companies are working to rebrand their toxic drugs and poisons into "well-tolerated" medications that somehow over time become "non-poisonous" or "cures" or are advertised to sound like supplements.

Would medical science prescribe a cancer causing drug to cancer patients? The answer to this question is indirectly given by Jim Morris in his 15 February 2005 *Washington Post* article titled *"What if the cure is also a cause?"*:

> Last March, the US federal government issued an unusually detailed alert to the nation's 5.5 million health care workers: the powerful drugs used in chemotherapy can themselves cause cancer and pose a risk to nurses, pharmacists and others who handle them.

Chemotherapy drugs in human and animal studies have shown they have the potential to cause cancer or reproductive problems, said Thomas Connor, a research biologist with the National Institute for Occupational Safety and Health (NIOSH).

Chemo-drugs, like radiation, generate huge amounts of the highly reactive hydroxyl radical that damages cell membranes and disrupts the electron transport system in cells as well as protein synthesis. Natural enzyme and micronutrient levels drop rapidly and that accelerates cell death. Such a new surge of free radicals is generated by chemo-drugs which are cytotoxic to cancer cells as well as normal cells. Thus many young normal cells die due to the treatment. Most of the known carcinogens, including benzene and at least 40 other toxic chemicals in cigarette smoke and pesticides generate free radicals that create oxidative stress in cells, impairing their aerobic respiration or damaging DNA and mitochondrial DNA, turning them into cancer cells. It is this very same toxicity that is common to carcinogens and chemotherapy-drugs. That's the reason why the aforementioned alert for carcinogenic cancer-drug came as no surprise.

Big Pharma is not about protecting or promoting your health. It is about exerting and extending control over all aspects of human health. The less control you have over your health, the more control they have over both you and your health. So how much control do they actually want? That depends on what and how the substance will impact the bottom line.

Britain is reviewing the laws on the regulation of tailored herbal treatments, but Dr. Canter wants them banned, even at the risk of a backlash from Chinese or Indian communities. In some countries doctors practice phytotherapy, which uses extracts from a single plant and closely follows the principles of pharmacology.[119]

So phytotherapy, using "extracts from a single plant" that "closely follow the principles of pharmacology" is all right, while individual attention from a herbalist is outright dangerous. If you recommend a glass of juice made of orange plus carrot plus red spinach with a spoon of coconut oil and if the health of the person improves and they also lose some fat, well there you go...it is a drug! Can you see how Codex is slowly taking control of your kitchen?

There is another grave danger. While allopathic medicine is moving towards individual customization, they want to take that principle away from nutritional interventions. Developments and research in therapeutic approaches that improve or restore health will be stifled if the principles of pharmacology are adopted as the only way to treat diseases and degenerative conditions in the human body. The mammalian biological system does not use pharmacological principles in generating an immune response or to activate cells that target pathogens or cancer cells, or in the production of antibodies or anti-pathogenic proteins such perforin, and neither in the repair of genetic material. When you legally only provide for pharmacological principles, you only create more drugs to be put into the human body. Such a law goes against the natural health processes of the human biological system. It only works towards the bottom line of pharmaceutical companies at the expense of health. Society and its productivity are dependent on health, not on the number of drugs or the amount of pharmaceutical benefit one gets. When a system of law is put in place that makes pharmacological principles the only system of treatment, we can say goodbye to the use of an orange or a lemon to cure scurvy. By then, it will be too good to own a pharmaceutical company but too late for mankind.

By then Codex would have given full control of all home remedies and your kitchen and orchard to Big Pharma. Can we change the course of the engines that are steaming in this direction? Big Pharma can bankroll what they choose and all you have is a deaf or illiterate congressman or parliamentarian. Bear in mind that lobbies against health have been very successful. Take for instance, coconut oil – your doctor or even your consultant dietician may tell you that it is bad for your heart because it contains cholesterol!

The point is that governments are no longer in control of health as the pharmaceutical agenda to promote pharmaceutical benefits is spreading like a bad cancer. Greed has become their god.

### c) Why doctors will give you only half-truths about...
### The War on Nature
Oxidative stress is implicated in most human diseases because the superoxide can oxidatively damage molecules in the mammalian biological system. These oxidatively-damaged molecules can initiate disease states. For instance, oxidatively-

damaged glucose and protein molecules form glycated proteins that can lead to cataracts etc. Oxidatively-damaged glucose molecules cannot form conjugates to enter cell walls and pass into the cell where they can be used to produce ATP. Also, oxidatively-damaged cell membranes lose their functional integrity that can lead to disease states. And there is a bigger problem with excess superoxide. Excess superoxide is the amount of superoxide that cannot be scavenged by the antioxidants or the antioxidant system in the cells and it can react with other useful molecules such as nitric oxide (NO) to produce the highly reactive secondary radical called the peroxynitrite radical that can damage cell membranes and lead to disease conditions such as cardiovascular disease, arthritis, ED etc. It is also well established that if the glutathione-catalase system cannot effectively convert hydrogen peroxide formed during cell metabolism, it can react with the excess superoxide to form the very deleterious hydroxyl radicals that can damage cell membranes, protein molecules, hormone molecules, enzyme molecules and even mtDNA and DNA molecules and lead to the development of a host of disease states and cancers.

The biochemical mechanisms that point to the role of free radicals in the development of disease states and cancers and degenerative conditions as well as in the progress of aging became clear over the last two decades of research and are now well understood. From an implication, free radicals and free radical reactions and free radical-induced reactions are now understood as the cause of many diseases pointing to the biochemical origin of disease other than caused by pathogens. The biochemically harmful effects of free radicals are real and measurable and are not "alleged harmful effects" as stated in a recent report in JAMA.[120]

Only natural antioxidants can effectively scavenge free radicals in the mammalian biological system and do it safely

The antioxidants in mammalian biological systems work in an

integrated network system. L-ascorbic acid can donate electrons to all the water-soluble antioxidant molecules in the system directly, a process that recharges or recycles them and it can also donate electrons to alpha-lipoic acid that can then donate electrons to both the water-soluble and fat-soluble antioxidant molecules of the mammalian biological system and any other natural antioxidant molecules (from food or edible sources) that can work within the natural antioxidant system of mammals. This is a critical factor in the antioxidant defense mechanism. Populations that consume a diet that offers natural antioxidant molecules from a variety of sources tend to have a lower risk of cardiovascular disease, arthritis, diabetes, hypertension and cancers. Hence, antioxidants from fruits, green leafy vegetables and fish oils and natural olive oil or sesame seed oil or coconut oil would prove to be better for health.

The mammalian biological system operates on the L-form antioxidants. These are antioxidants found in natural sources, excepting olive oil which occurs in the D-form in nature. Free radical biochemistry is harmful and can produce deleterious and lethal effects over time whereas natural antioxidants scavenge free radicals and prevent or minimize the harmful effects of free radical biochemistry in the body. That is not difficult to understand but there is another interesting point about antioxidants.

The healthy biochemical pathways of the mammalian biological system operating on L-form antioxidants involve the production and utilization of ATP molecules, production of antibodies, collagen, melatonin, hormones and other useful biomolecules – all of them dependent on antioxidant-driven biochemical processes that can be disrupted by excess free radicals. In such a system, the antioxidant molecules that donate electrons during the scavenging activity become "spent" but remain stable and may either be recharged and recycled for further scavenging activity or may be broken down and utilized in the synthesis of other useful biomolecules. For instance, L-ascorbic acid may be converted into collagen with the help of colloidal copper or colloidal gold after it is "spent".

Natural antioxidants, therefore, actually prevent the development of disease states by preventing oxidative stress by excess free radicals and by preventing the development of secondary radicals. Otherwise, they decrease or diminish oxidative damage and its harmful effects. Now there is interest in tapping the potential of natural antioxidants from food or edible sources for inducing and promoting rapid free radical scavenging activity to study the antioxidant-driven effects for reversing the cellular and biochemical damage of excess.

Many people are taking antioxidant supplements to supplement the natural antioxidant intake from their diet to improve the free radical scavenging activity in their bodies as a way to prevent health problems and prevent the development of disease states or otherwise to slow down the aging process or slow down the progression of disease conditions that are free-radical induced. Yet, the authors of the report in JAMA titled "Mortality in Randomized Trials of Antioxidant Supplements for Primary and Secondary Prevention Systematic Review and Meta-analysis" are not sure when they state "whether antioxidant supplements are beneficial or harmful is uncertain."

Many primary or secondary prevention trials of antioxidant supplements have been conducted to prevent several diseases. They conclude that "antioxidant supplements, with the potential exception of selenium, were without significant effects on gastrointestinal cancers and increased all-cause mortality."

The methodological quality of some of the trials was assessed using the published reports, which may not reflect the actual design and bias risk of the trials. Some authors responded to our requests for further information. All available nonenzymatic antioxidants work differently in the human body and most of them exert effects that are nonantioxidant. We are not able to point to the specific biochemical mechanisms behind the detrimental effects.[121]

They performed adjusted-rank vitamin C; vitamin A and vitamin C; vitamin C and vitamin E; vitamin E and selenium; selenium and zinc; beta-carotene, vitamin C, and vitamin E; beta-carotene, vitamin C, vitamin E, and selenium; beta-carotene, vitamin C, vitamin E, selenium, and zinc; vitamin A, vitamin C, vitamin E, selenium, and zinc; vitamin A, vitamin C, vitamin E, selenium, methionine, and ubiquinone. In 11 trials, participants were supplemented with different mixtures of antioxidants as well as with vitamins and minerals without antioxidant properties.

The fact is that most antioxidants in the mammalian biological system also work in a synergistic fashion. For instance, L-ascorbic acid recycles melatonin and enhances its effects threefold. Melatonin is a brain-body antioxidant that has anticancer effects, primarily due to its ability to donate electrons to both the lipid and non-lipid part of the cell wall. This biochemical repair restores cell wall integrity and that in turn promotes aerobic respiration and consequently prevents the cell wall from acquiring a strong positive charge {positive cell membrane potential (CMP)} a key factor in the transformation from aerobic respiration to anaerobic respiration which initiates the formation of cancer cells.

It has been suggested that antioxidant supplements may show interdependency and may have effects only if given in combination.[122] That is clearly a logical suggestion within the working of the mammalian biological system and the fact that the natural antioxidant molecules work in an integrated fashion in a network and also in synergistic roles. Most of the studies on vitamins are designed around the administration of one vitamin and many of these studies use analogues or synthetics instead of the L-form molecules from food sources.

Synthetic vitamins are like any other synthetic molecules, but because of their antioxidant nature they are able to donate one electron, after which they do not remain stable but are broken down in a metabolic process that yields hydrogen peroxide. Administering synthetic vitamins in persons with disease states can thus be counterproductive. These people already have a problem associated with or directly caused by excess free radicals, including hydroxyl radicals. Adding substances into their biological system that can lead to the formation or more hydroxyl radicals only exacerbates their free radical biochemistry. There are several studies that show that synthetic vitamins are harmful. For a therapeutic purpose, there is a need to enhance the free radical scavenging potential in patients with disease states that successfully converts all the hydroxyl radicals and hydrogen peroxide into water and oxygen as soon as they are formed – something that occurs during the prime of youth.

The aim of the review in the JAMA study[123] was to analyze the effects of antioxidant supplements (beta-carotene, vitamins A and E, vitamin C [ascorbic acid], and selenium) on all-cause mortality of adults included in primary and secondary prevention trials. The authors "found that antioxidant supplements, with the potential exception of selenium, were without significant effects on gastrointestinal cancers and increased all-cause mortality." That would be quite the natural expectation if synthetic antioxidants were used as supplements in patients with cancers. Cancer patients have high amounts of excess superoxide and a large number of hydroxyl radicals.

Several new review studies on nutrients, called meta-analysis, seem to contradict either what we know from previous research, or what our intelligence tells us should be true. You only have to scan the headlines and pay attention to the "newly found" dangers of this or that natural substance. From St. John's Wort to Kava Kava, from vitamin C to vitamin E, we hear that they are "not effective" or worse – that they may be dangerous.

We know one fundamental truth – and that is nutrition and

nutritional intake through food is what makes us grow and is essential for health. And we also know that by increasing our natural antioxidant intake through supplements made from food substances, but not in undue excess, we increase the free radical scavenging potential in our bodies and tend to improve health. That is basic health science or food science. Yet a new field of study called meta-analysis may be used to discredit the role and function of natural supplements or does it prove one fact very bluntly – synthetic vitamins are harmful.

*Fish oils "don't work"?*

On March 24 , 2006, the British Medical Journal published a meta-analysis (a study of other studies) on omega-3 fatty acids that prompted headlines around the world to the effect that "fish oils don't work." This is not the first time a meta-analysis has triggered headlines that discredit natural health supplements. These meta-analyses are a funny piece of work that is made out to look like sophisticated science, probably targeted at laypeople. Dr. Robert Verkerk, of the Alliance for Natural Health, says those studies are manipulated. This is a new kind of study that is highly regarded these days, but it is based on a choose-and-pick approach where older studies are reviewed and analyzed to combine their wisdom. The criteria of inclusion/exclusion of previous studies in the analysis, and the decision of how to give different weights to different results are so rubbery that almost any conclusion becomes possible. One of the more recent studies that attempts to trash nutrients takes on the health benefits of fish oils... and may be used to coincide with a launch of a synthetic ...making such studies more of a marketing gimmick rather than a real scientific study.

And such a coincidence has indeed happened. The fact that the meta-analysis throwing doubt on omega-3 fish oils coincides with the launch of a pharmaceutical version of the same type of fats made by chemical giant Solvay and it reminds me of the tryptophan disaster of more than a decade ago.

In meta-analyses there is a big catch, like a mathematical fallacy in which one tries to divide by zero. The "trick" lies in assessing "all-cause mortality". Take for instance, the study on vitamin E. The overall conclusion that high-dose vitamin E causes increased mortality could also have been a statistical artifact, with no biological relevance. Since the study assessed all-cause mortality, and not just cardiovascular mortality, any other cause of mortality is included. Other factors could easily have contributed to the greater death rate in the higher dose vitamin E group found when trials were pooled. The pooling of risks to mortality creates the desired warp and twisting. It is a strange science.

Meta-analysis can make a nutrient into a factor that increases mortality or it can "show" that beta-carotene, vitamin A and other antioxidant vitamins such as vitamin E are harmful. It can make people doubt the benefits of omega-3 oils by making headlines like "fish oils don't work." On the other hand, it can be used to investigate the effect on heart disease risk of a Unilever margarine enriched with alpha-linolenic acid (ALA), an important short-chain omega-3 found to be rich in Mediterranean diets, well known for its health promoting properties, and conclude clearly the beneficial effects of ALA-enriched margarine on reducing heart disease risk! In one meta-analysis, scientists can decry a natural antioxidant that promotes heart health, while in another it can promote the same class of natural antioxidant in a hydrogenated oil that introduces trans-fatty acids into the bloodstream as circulating fatty acids that promote plaque formation and heart disease and damage cell walls. A fishy tool that can be well adapted as a basis for promo-tional literature and published in peer review journals for marketing synthetic products unless the consumer knows the real science of natural antioxidants and their biochemical function in free radical biochemistry. But it is the headlines that influence consumer behavior rather than the research in scientific journals. Few read the actual studies.

*Antioxidant omega-3 oils in cardiovascular disease*

Dr. Alexander Leaf, a professor and his team of scientists at Harvard, had done extensive work on omega-3 fish oils and documented the beneficial effects of this natural oil on health and cardiovascular disease, and an experiment was designed to prove its antiarrythmic role. Leaf and other researchers cultured neonatal heart cells from rats. Under the microscope, these cells clumped together which as a clump of heart cells beat spontaneously and rhythmically just like the heart as an organ. Toxic agents known to produce fatal arrhythmias in humans were added to the medium bathing the cultured cells, and the effects of adding the omega-3 fatty acids were observed. Increased extracellular Ca2+, the cardiac glycoside ouabain, isoproterenol, lysophosphatidylcholine and acylcarnitine, thromboxane, and even the Ca2+ ionophore A23187 were tested. All of these agents induced tachyarrhythmias in the isolated myocytes.[124]

Of particular interest are the effects of elevated perfusate Ca2+ and ouabain on the myocytes. Both agents induced rapid contractions, contractures and fibrillation of the myocytes. When EPA was added to the superfusate, the beating rate slowed, and when the high Ca2+ or ouabain was added in the presence of the EPA, no arrhythmia was induced. Furthermore, after a violent fibrillation was induced in the cells by both elevated calcium and ouabain, addition of EPA stopped the arrhythmias, and the cells resumed their fairly regular contractions. The addition of the dilapidated BSA to remove the free fatty acid from the myocytes resulted in recurrence of the arrhythmia.

This indicated two important facts as outlined by Dr. Leaf. First, the EPA could be extracted from the cells in the continued presence of the toxins, and the arrhythmia would return, which indicated that the fatty acids were acting without strong ionic or covalent binding to any constituent in the cell membrane. If they had such binding, we would not have been able to extract the EPA from the cells with the albumin. It appears the free fatty acids act directly on the heart cells and need only partition (dissolve) into the hospitable hydrophobic interior of phospholipids of the plasma membranes of myocytes to elicit their antiarrhythmic actions. Second, when we tested the ethyl ester of the EPA, it had no prompt antiarrhythmic action; only the free fatty acid with its negative carboxyl charge was antiarrhythmic. Herein lies the key in understanding the role of omega-3 oil – its role as an antioxidant. Another study reported in the Annals of Internal Medicine concluded that omega-3 fatty acids can slow the course of atherosclerosis and may reduce the risk of further heart disease. Many studies have come to a similar conclusion.

After several population studies that noted the positive effects of omega-3 fish oils and laboratory evidence, I explained their role as an antioxidant in an article. Now, it was within mainstream science and the growing understanding and popularity of natural biomolecules that are integrated into normal and healthy cellular function and at the same time more people have became aware of drug toxicities, I was expecting "studies" to contradict omega-3 fish oil studies, but I expected something subtle like casting a doubt at first and then discrediting it. I did not expected a foolhardy and blatant "fish oils don't work" in a British Medical Journal.

The fact remains that natural omega-3 fish oil, like many other natural oils are antioxidants that scavenge free radicals in the cell wall and biomembranes and provide an electron to the lipid part of the molecules in biomembranes, that was lost to a free radical and that restores stability and functional integrity to the biomembranes. That sums up, in a nutshell, the antioxidant role of such oils (and) fat soluble antioxidants in restoring healthy function of cells and tissues. These natural antioxidants are an integral part of our evolutionary history whereas synthetic molecules are not.

Please note the use of synthetic vitamin E in the Miller study, and this could have explained the negative results found by Miller et al,[125] as well as those found earlier by Dr. Marc Penn and colleagues from the Cleveland Clinic, published in The Lancet. Again, note the negative results from a very small clutch of studies on synthetic vitamins like synthetic beta-carotene and vitamin E, which were administered to diseased or high risk subjects. These authors asserted that beta-carotene, vitamin A and other antioxidant vitamins such as vitamin E were harmful. That conclusion in The Lancet, by Dr. Penn and his colleagues, is correct and wholly supports what we have been saying – that synthetic molecules are harmful and cannot be incorporated into therapies and diet. Synthetic biomolecules can suppress the immune system or disrupt the production of natural antioxidants in the body or disrupt normal biochemical pathways in the body, a problem mediated through the production of hydrogen peroxide during the cell metabolic breakdown of synthetics under oxidative stress leading to the formation of more hydroxyl radicals. So, while L-ascorbic acid intake improves collagen formation in the body and improves elasticity of blood vessels, the D-form may produce bleeding in patients.

*Synthetic antioxidants for smokers*
The report of the study in Finland of Vitamin E and beta-carotene on the incidence of cancer in male smokers is important because it drives home the message that vitamins may increase cancer.[126] Synthetic vitamins, that is. Synthetic vitamins are not food. They are synthetic chemicals. Only vitamins from dietary sources or edible plants can be considered nutrients for the body.

The first study in question was the 1994 Alpha-Tocopherol Beta-Carotene Cancer Prevention Study (ATBC) involving Finnish men who were heavy smokers and alcohol drinkers. The volunteers were either given 20 milligrams of synthetic beta-

134

carotene, vitamin E, a combination of the two, or a placebo. The expected outcome suggested that there was an 18% increase in lung cancer rates in the beta-carotene only group. Cigarette smoke contains about 4000 toxic chemicals, of which 40 are known carcinogens. The metabolic breakdown of synthetic chemicals and alcohol yields toxic metabolites that yield the superoxide radical and hydrogen peroxide. Similarly, the breakdown of synthetic beta-carotene and synthetic vitamin E also results in the same biochemical problem in the liver and that simply adds to creating excess free radicals and oxidative stress from hydroxyl radicals. Hydroxyl radicals can cause damage to membranes and DNA molecules and transform normal cells into cancer cells. In other words, synthetics accelerate free radical biochemistry.

The second trial was the 1996 Carotenoid and Retinol Efficacy Trial (CARET), which was a lung cancer prevention study involving a combination of 30 mg of synthetic beta-carotene and 25,000 iu of retinol (synthetic formed vitamin A) versus placebo. The volunteers were either smokers or asbestos workers. This study was stopped early due to the fact that preliminary findings suggested that there was a 28% increase in cancer rates in the beta-carotene/vitamin A group, compared to placebo. Asbestos in the human body can create biochemical problems. The findings in this study are consistent with the expectation of higher rates of cancers as would be with all other studies that test synthetics. The correct conclusion is that synthetic vitamins contribute to free radical biochemistry in the human biological system and in people who introduce other substances into the body that also generate free radicals, the risk of generating hydroxyl radicals increases while in some people it becomes excess, leading to the development of cancers. Much of the outcome depends on the intake of antioxidants from dietary sources.

The most critical fact that deserves special scrutiny in the

Finnish studies is that the beta-carotene and vitamins used in these studies are synthetic and not from dietary sources. It is interesting to note that dietary intake of various antioxidants, such as carbonyl from broccoli or olive oil, other carotenoids (such as lycopene and cryptoxanthin) is far more strongly associated with lower cancer risk while intake of synthetic antioxidants tend to raise that risk, especially in smokers and those who consume alcohol or those who are already have cancers in them.

### Recycling vs. metabolic breakdown

People who have cancers and those who smoke and consume alcohol, in general, have lower levels of natural vitamin C. That by itself is a compromising factor for the immune function of white blood cells and T4 cells. These lower levels of natural vitamin C are insufficient to fully recycle other antioxidants directly or through alpha-lipoic acid. Recycling the fat-soluble antioxidants through alpha-lipoic acid becomes critical in cancer patients because of the greater amounts of fat-soluble antioxidants required to biochemically repair the cell membranes (by donating electrons and reducing their positive potential) in order to restore their functional integrity. And natural vitamin C cannot recycle synthetic vitamins. The synthetic vitamins are targeted for metabolic breakdown once they have donated their electrons.

Natural molecules, such as natural oils, fat-soluble antioxidants and natural vitamins have been part of the mammalian diet for 65 million years and primate diets for 15 million years of hominid evolution. We read in our primary schools how effective vitamin C was in curing scurvy in sailors. Research in free radical science has already contributed so much knowledge to mainstream science. Yet we have researchers who dare state that natural antioxidants "don't work" and are harmful while synthetic molecules work and are safer?

*History of science is important*
History of the use of oils is a part of that history as well as part of the history of marketing. A few decades ago, a particular association began lobbying and commenced a media campaign against natural tropical oils saying that these oils are highly saturated. Their campaign was designed to get people to switch to vegetable oils that they did not say were, in fact, hydrogenated oils. In the body, these long-chain fatty acids become converted to circulating lipoproteins and hence contribute to the artery-clogging factor. Their campaign succeeded, in spite of the fact that tropical oils are not long-chain fatty acids but are medium-chain fatty acids which are readily broken down in the liver to produce energy, do not become circulating fat molecules and do not contribute to artery-clogging. Other positive information on medium-chain fatty acids was never brought to light, including their anti-inflammatory properties and that they are used by the body to produce antimicrobial and antiviral molecules and have cardio-protective functions, as well as that they may be used to synthesize other molecules that have anti-inflammatory or antibacterial properties.

The success of that campaign against tropical oils contributed to rising rates of obesity, cardiovascular disease and cancers and created an expanded market for a wider range of drugs.

It can be speculated that, as a general rule, the synthetic oil starts as a prescriptory medication in order to gain a foothold in the market and that later it may be 'moved' into the supplement category to broaden its market. However, the war on natural fish oil is being fought differently. Meta-studies appear to be used as a tool to discredit the natural oil which is already part of the diet as well as other scientific works in reputable journals for purposes of possibly altering consumer buying behavior in favor of the synthetic oil.

People are more educated than before and too many people know how science is manipulated. These people will not put "prescriptory health" above natural health. Health is a result of nutrients from food sources and it cannot be an outcome of prescriptions that contain synthetics or analogues. Consumers should know the difference between the two. This points to the need to improve science literacy in Congress and Parliament, and the need to scrutinize the media that attempt to promote synthetic stuff as superior and better than natural biomolecules, while at the same time discrediting other scientific studies that prove or note the beneficial function of natural biomolecules in the human body. It also points to the need for a sound health education in primary and secondary schools and as a subsidiary subject in colleges and universities.

# Chapter 5

# Psychodictatorship

*Psychiatry means the medicine of the soul. Yet, in most of its applied forms it possesses no soul. And it can hardly be called a science. It is not facts and theories. It is either about only facts or only theories. There is a huge unabridged gap in psychiatry and this gap constantly generates social controversies and scientific contradictions*

## a) Why doctors will give you only half-truths about...
### The Pseudoscience of Psychiatry

Sigmund Freud had without a doubt an important impact on the history and evolution of Western civilization and ideas, fertilizing it with insightful observations about the human "psyche". On the other hand, the patriarch of psychoanalysis established a long line of dominant masculine therapists and theorists, strengthened and scientificized phallocracy and founded intentionally or unintentionally a psychoanalytic cult, a dedicated "hermetic" brotherhood of specialists.

Under Freud, women were turned from complete human beings to malformed, imperfect and inherently inhibited versions of man. Penis envy, how more phallocratic can it get?

It is no wonder that every year an average of 10 psychiatrists are expelled from the American Psychiatric Association for sexual misconduct with a patient.[127] The therapist pretty much like the confessor are supposed to be patriarchal figures, free of sexual "sin" and projections, free of the "beast inside", all forgiving, all understanding, bestowed with the power to "restore". Nothing could be further from reality. With few exceptions, most of the time it is about force, the power to violate, to control the inner human, to manipulate one's psychological

context. It is a confidence game that when successful is trans-
ferred from the couch or the confessional to society at large, a
power game that is exploiting the dehumanization of interper-
sonal or social relations and the gaps created by anti-humanitarian policies, behaviors and perceptions, another case of trust
parasitism. As Jeffrey Mason commented, *"What we need are more
kindly friends and fewer professionals."*[128]

Freud presented some arguments that were philosophical and
not scientific, and concocted them with mythological figures that
were analyzed completely out of context with their historical
origins and their semantics. Oedipus, for example, in the ancient
world has probably never been perceived as someone governed
by a patricidal sex drive. The Oedipus tragedy revolves around
power, and succession of power. The ancient Greek world did not
need to make any sexual insinuations as sex was clearly and
freely present in myth, speech and everyday life. Freud's interpretation is just a product of a more taboo-burdened era and
Freud possibly distorted the Oedipus figure to relieve his own
obsessions:

> His destiny moves us only because it might have been ours –
> because the oracle laid the same curse upon us before our
> birth as upon him. It is the fate of all of us, perhaps, to direct
> our first sexual impulse towards our mother and our first
> hatred and our first murderous wish against our father. Our
> dreams convince us that this is so.[129]

And elsewhere,

> I found in myself a constant love for my mother, and jealousy
> of my father. I now consider this to be a universal event in
> childhood.

A man's obsession, an era in science. Freud projected his personal experiences and obsessions onto society and science, and that is a typical example of *transference*. His ideas were more philosophical than scientific. Yet, a "scientific" discipline was created from them. If the Freudian Oedipus interpretation was of any scientific potency, it would be expected that in the rather taboo-free animal state patricidal species could and would be found in abundance...

There could be no better critique on Freudian science than the comment himself made on philosophy and science:

Philosophy is not opposed to science, it behaves itself as if it were a science, and to a certain extent it makes use of the same methods; but it parts company with science, in that it clings to the illusion that it can produce a complete and coherent picture of the universe, though in fact that picture must needs fall to pieces with every new advance in our knowledge. Its methodological error lies in the fact that it over-estimates the epistemological value of our logical operations, and to a certain extent admits the validity of other sources of knowledge, such as intuition.[130]

Indeed, that is exactly what Freud and his followers did: they admitted the validity of Freud's intuition.

What resulted was not a psychological philosophy but rather a pseudoscience. It could not be tested, verified, falsified, or create prognosis.

Karl Popper himself attributed to psychoanalysis characteristics of a pseudoscience. The great philosopher of science declared that:

...Thus what worried me was neither the problem of truth, at that stage at least, nor the problem of exactness or measurability. It was rather that I felt that these other three theories, though posing as science, had in fact more in common with primitive myths than with science; that they resembled astrology rather than astronomy.

I found that those of my friends, who were admirers of Marx, Freud, and Adler, were impressed by a number of points common to these theories, and especially by their apparent *explanatory power*. These theories appear to be able to explain practically everything that happened within the fields to which they referred. The study of any of them seemed to have the effect of an intellectual conversion or revelation, opening your eyes to a new truth hidden from those not yet initiated. Once your eyes were thus opened you saw confirmed instances everywhere: the world was full of *verifications* of the theory. Whatever happened always confirmed it. Thus its truth appeared manifest; and unbelievers were clearly people who did not want to see the manifest truth; who refuse to see it, either because it was against their class interest, or because of their repressions which were still "unanalyzed" and crying aloud for treatment...

...The two psycho-analytic theories were in a different class. They were simply non-testable, irrefutable. There was no conceivable human behavior which could contradict them. This does not mean that Freud and Adler were not seeing certain things correctly; I personally do not doubt that much of what they say is of considerable importance, and may well play its part one day in a psychological science which is testable. But it does mean that those "clinical observations" which analysts naively believe confirm their theory cannot do this any more than the daily confirmations which astrologers find in their practice. And as for Freud's epic of the Ego, the Super-ego, and the Id, no substantially stronger claim to scientific status can be made for it than for Homer's collected stories from Olympus. These theories describe some facts, but in the manner of myths. They contain most interesting psychological suggestions, but not in a testable form.[131]

Again, a science was created by admitting the validity of Freud's intuitions...

Something more compact, more science-like was needed than the loose connotations of psychoanalysis. And it appeared in the form of behaviorism, a discipline that would study the behavior of living creatures and their response to stimuli to decide of the rules that governed or at least permeated the Self. Though, without a doubt, useful and fruitful observations derived from behavioral psychology, it could not stand on its own as a science. Behaviorism suffered from the exact opposite birth defect of psychoanalysis: while psychoanalysis suffered from lack of raw data and precise scientific terminology, behaviorism suffered from the lack of an underlying theory or even a philosophy. Behaviorism is like Douglas Adams' Deep Thought, a super computer created by a supra-intelligent race that was fed every available data to come up with The Answer to the Ultimate Question of Life, the Universe, and Everything. And it did. The answer was 42 and it was without a doubt the Correct answer. The only problem was now that the sentient creatures possessed the answer to everything, they had to create an even more evolved Hyper-computer to find out what the correct question to The Answer was.[132]

Behavioral psychology was psychiatry's 42. And the question to the answer psychiatry's Big Brains came up with was the Brain Itself. Mental disorders were interpreted as dysfunctions of the Brain, as biochemical disturbances. And if brain biochemistry was the problem, then chemistry would have to be the solution. Thus the chemical warfare against the brain was reasoned and, thus, tons of neuromodulating chemical compounds were unleashed onto the mentally ill or the dysfunctional. Or the weird. Or the saddened. Or the unreasonably active. Or the sleepless. Or the frustrated. Or the lazy. Or the angry. Or the unfit. Once there was the scientific argument to back up the necessity of psychodrugs, the question of who would be institutionalized, or chemically assaulted, drugged, regulated and controlled was left to experts and their opinions. Being crazy became not a condition but, rather, a definition. People who are deemed crazy are crazy by definition.

And who better in definitions than the DSM, the Statistical Manual of Mental Disorders, the mosaic law of mental disorders?

The DSM classification is a prejudiced invention, a biased pseudoscientific concoction. In a way it is a contract, an arrangement, a settlement between psychiatrists, authorities and society determining who is equal enough to live among us without chemical regulation or psychiatric intervention or institutionalization. It is a mental cleansing, a mental Hygiene program in the same manner that the Nazi's had their Racial Hygiene and ethnic cleansing program.

It is not scientific. Mental illness is determined in a behavioristic fashion. It is shaped by the existing social prejudices: you can find no "obsessive TV viewing disorder", no "football fanatic disorder", no "obsessive success impulse" or "obsessive conformism disorder". These conditions are all agreed upon and even imposed by modern societies. The more a behavior is accepted or well tolerated by a society, the less it is susceptible to being classified as disorder. It is not about science or health care. It is more about social norms. It is about the unfit and the intolerable. It is about consensus. It is about social and scientific consensus.

Psychologist Renée Garfinkel described the fashion after which disorders and diagnostic criteria are agreed upon, the fashion after the context of mental segregation is reached, the genesis of the DSM:

The low level of intellectual effort was shocking. Diagnoses were developed by majority vote on the level we would use to choose a restaurant. You feel like Italian, I feel like Chinese, so let's go to a cafeteria. Then it's typed into the computer. It may reflect on our naiveté, but it was our belief that there would be an attempt to look at things scientifically.[133]

That doesn't sound at all scientific. It sounds lobbyist, it reflects a guild mentality. Unfortunately, this kind of consensus has a huge social impact. Psychiatric consensus, when not confronted or checked by common sense, establishes a self-serving diagnostic and treatment regime.

One of the leading behaviorists was B.F. Skinner. Skinner argued that free will and dignity are mere delusions. In his own words : "The fundamental mistake made by all those who choose weak methods of control is to assume that the balance of control is left to the individual, when in fact it is left to other conditions."[134] Psychiatry was not willing to succumb to this mistake. It would divide and conquer, define and control. Skinner's argument a lot of times seems to be the ultimate goal of psychiatric intervention: Negate free will, destroy dignity. The mental patient has to conform to the psychiatric instructions and reform. He has to accept his weakness to handle his own condition, agree to the doctor's suggestion that he is not well and only when he admits defeat and surrenders himself to the intentions of the psychiatrist can he hope to return to what's left of his former life. It is a game of power, of admitting your weakness, of recognizing superiority and control of others over your own life. It is about authority, submission, conformism and reform. It is the mental inquisition, it is McCarthyism, it is totalitarianism, it is the Troika. As Skinner's book title suggested, it is "Beyond freedom and dignity". It is the psychiatric regime in which, as Thomas Szasz described: "Joy and sadness, fear and elation, anger, greed—all human aspirations and passions—are thus interpreted as the manifestations of unintentional, amoral, biochemical processes. In such a world nothing is willed; everything happens."

And this is exactly what made a disillusioned and frustrated psychiatrist, Loren Mosher, vow and protest that he wanted "...

no part of a psychiatry of oppression and social control."[135]

This behaviorist vision of a world urged by the most notable psychologists of the 20th century, Carl Rogers to warn us that: "We can choose to use our growing knowledge to enslave people in ways never dreamed of before, depersonalizing them, controlling them by means so carefully selected that they will never be aware of their loss of personhood."

Of course sometimes drug intervention might be necessary to help some people when they are way over their heads. Of course some professionals who can understand and sympathize with the human condition should be available to resort to it. But psychiatry, in most of its current expressions, and most of the time, is not about offering help to those in need. It is about power, submission and segregation, it is about chemical punishment, it is about creating armies of drug addicts and pathetic puppets. Most of the time, it is not about helping people regain power and control over their own lives. It is about disempowerment, it is about creating an overall feeling of weakness and worthlessness and complete addiction to the psychiatric universe. Exceptions of notable, worthy and helpful mental health professionals are not rare. But they can't possibly make up for the threat that the psychiatric establishment as a whole poses to civil liberties, to free will, to freedom of speech and to democracy itself.

Who are we kidding? For the most of the Western world, animals are castrated to get them off our streets, people are chemically or legally imprisoned. We rename people with special needs people with special skills and toss them into special schools. God, they must feel so special after such special treatment. Everything we don't like we eliminate or hide under the luxurious carpet of social welfare to get it out of our sight. This is not a civilized social welfare, this is a farewell to civilized society, a disguised regression to brutality.

And it is all about symptoms, treat symptoms, cure symptoms, disguise symptoms, hide them, wear a heavy layer of makeup. From somatic medicine to psychiatry, from politics to society all we learn, all we do is to treat symptoms and not the causes. We are shallow.

Brighter future societies will hold us accountable for crimes against our fellow men in the same manner that we are condemning inhuman practices of the past. We are so accustomed to our cruelty that we believe that we are morally superior and kind.

We must understand. We must change. Psychiatry must change.

It is time for the reformist to reform into a kind and loving companion of humanity instead of a cruel tyrant.

### b) Why doctors will give you only half-truths about...
### Depression

It can be as crippling as a car crash. It can be life threatening. It can be torturing. Depression accounts for a 3.4% of total disability and premature loss of life in developed countries in women and 1.3% in men.[136] A projective study estimated that by the year 2020 major unipolar depression will be the second leading cause of disability-adjusted life years (DALYs), surpassed only by ischemic heart disease and supplanting road-traffic accidents.[137]

Depression can be deadly. Up to 15% of patients suffering from unipolar depression eventually commit suicide.[138]

So, what it is actually going on? Why are people so heavily burdened by this mood disorder?

It is all biochemistry, the proponents of chemical intervention will profess pompously. Of course it is. Who can deny our biochemical substrate? But who is also foolish enough to deny the way society and lifestyle affects both our emotional and mental state?

Loren Mosher was one of the few to point out the limitations of a reductionist, mechanistic, chemical psychiatry both on patients and practitioners:

> These psychopharmacological limitations on our abilities to be complete physicians also limit our intellectual horizons. No longer do we seek to understand whole persons in their social contexts – rather we are there to realign our patients' neurotransmitters. The *problem* is that it is very difficult to have a relationship with a neurotransmitter – whatever its configuration. So, our guild organization provides a rationale, by its neurobiological tunnel vision, for keeping our distance from the molecule conglomerates we have come to define as patients. We condone and promote the widespread use and misuse of toxic chemicals that we know have serious long-term effects – tardive dyskinesia, tardive dementia and serious withdrawal syndromes. So, do I want to be a drug company patsy who treats molecules with their formulary? No, thank you very much... It saddens me that after 35 years as a psychiatrist I look forward to being dissociated from such an organization (APA). In no way does it represent my interests. It is not within my capacities to buy into the current biomedical-reductionistic model heralded by the psychiatric leadership as once again marrying us to somatic medicine. This is a matter of fashion, politics and, like the pharmaceutical house connection, money."[139]

It must have been really painful for Mosher to resign. But sometimes painful choices are dictated by moral imperatives. The issue of pain and suffering is of great scientific and social significance.

Avoiding pain has always been a universal strategy for life and most of the time it has been highly successful. Pain informs us of something wrong or dangerous inside of us or close to us. It is desirable for societies and individuals to avoid pain. But not to turn a blind eye to it.

Modern societies do not overcome pain. They overlook it, they circumvent it, exile it, ban it. Images of healthy, successful, painless people were implanted in our psyche by the mass media brainwashing machines. And that was a deadly mistake for our civilization's progress. Yes we have to avoid pain, but a lower threshold of pain must be allowed so that we can understand it, understand its content and its value as an inherent alarm that allows us to sympathize with those in pain. The experience of pain is almost universal among sentient beings. It is a kind of universal language: it is immediately understood without the need to be translated or interpreted. We have to understand pain, at least at a minimum level, to be able to deploy strategies to avoid it. We immediately sympathize with people who are suffering because we know what it feels like. We are instantly motivated to ease their pain as we would like for our fellow man to do exactly the same thing for us: ease our pain. In the Greek language the word compassion is Sym-poneia, sympathize is sym-ponw, that is feel pain with someone or feel somebody else's pain. Pain is a universal human condition; to feel compassion is one of the qualities that makes us human. Now, societies today are suffering from anhedonia: that is we are unable to draw pleasure. They are also suffering from apathy: we are unable to act according to our emotions or even feel them. We have become intolerant to pain and incapable of joy, we have become desensualized, buried in our robotic lives, unable to correlate to anything else except profit and material possessions. It is obvious that the human psyche has been derailed and confused and that we have replaced its symbols, its functions and desires with poor substitutes. This is the imbalance that depression statistics depict, not an increase in the number of chemically-imbalanced people, but an imbalance of the very essence of the human entity and its societies. And alas, we are trying to deal with the imbalance created by virtuality, artificiality and the incorporation of substitutes in our innerverse and social surroundings by introducing chemical substitutes of pleasure and harmony and calm into our bodily chemistry, favoring artificiality and addiction even more, denying the organism the ability to restore itself!

We have not eliminated pain, we have just swept it under the carpet. Abuse of painkillers, abuse of sedatives, abuse of antidepressants. Physical pain has a lot in common with emotional pain. But there is a huge difference. In emotional pain, the pain can increase disproportionally to the cause that originally initiated it. It is a loop, a positive feedback effect endlessly increasing pain. It is like shouting in a canyon that I am in pain, or I am worthless, and hearing my own voice echoing indefinitely. This positive feedback loop cannot be intercepted by chemicals. Instead it is replaced with the positive feedback of receptor familiarization, of chemical or emotional dependency and addiction.

When it comes to emotional pain, whether it is described as a disorder or as a natural reaction to stimuli, it is our duty, as individuals and societies, to mitigate it, to offer a helping hand, to embrace the person in pain with love, understanding, compassion. A specialist should be our last resort when everything else fails. We have surrendered too much of our individual and social power, too many of our moral and ethical responsibilities to impersonal, faceless systems. We have actually dismantled the social fiber and everything that connects us. Who has time to deal with the human adventure or the human tragedy? Leave it to the experts, that's what they are trained for, that's what they are paid for. Alone and lost, in our times of need, we have to face a system that has become narcissist, self-regulated, self-determined, self-serving and thus, more often than not, indifferent, cruel and inhuman.

Why should a human creature feel of any value in a world that has abolished real value and replaced it with substitutes, stocks, material possessions, sexual connotations and virtually-induced excitement? How can he overcome pain when no one gives a damn? In a globalized world, the individual has become an isolated island nation that, under the weight of its unrealized potential for love and understanding, is sinking further and further down, an Atlantis that will never be notable enough to be mentioned or remembered. People are either raw materials or trash. They are not considered people anymore.

If the social context and the perceptions that are governing our civilization don't become more pragmatistic and humanistic, if they don't shift away from this utopia of virtuality and the senseless financial race to nowhere, then we will have to face the consequences. We are going to have to deal with a new breed of humans that will be dissociated from anything and will be unable to draw pleasure, understand pain, who will unable to feel.

What are we going to treat them with then?

Psychiatry has a long history of wrongful, barbaric and criminal "treatments" to exhibit, often displaying complete disregard to individuals, their vulnerability, their condition and further more their health, their dignity, their personality. From the surgical amputation called Lobotomy, to electroconvulsive therapy, psychiatry has often exercised, defended, imposed and boasted for anti-scientific, anti-humanitarian practices. Instead, from an open-minded "liberator" of the troubled, it literally opened other people's minds, acting like a totalitarian tormentor of the weak, the defenseless, the reactionary, the unfit and the intolerable. Mental hygiene has often become the banner of psycho-fascism.

Back then they were "fixing" the abnormal mind by operating on it. Now they say they "fix" chemical imbalance. Back then the commendable therapy was the lobotomy, a surgical procedure that disabled people for life, now it is the SSRIs.

All would be well, it would be just great, a real triumph of life sciences if the SSRIs actually did what they promised. But this hardly seems to be the case. In a 1998 meta-analysis of 19 double-blind clinical trials, Kirsch and Sapirstein concluded that:

> The data reviewed in this meta-analysis lead to a confident estimate that the response to inert placebos is approximately 75% of the response to active antidepressant medication. Whether the remaining 25% of the drug response is a true pharmacologic effect or an enhanced placebo effect cannot yet be determined, because of the relatively small number of studies in which active and inactive placebos have been compared.[140]

Ten years later Kirsch returned to the topic of the actual and not the suggested, proposed, promoted or advertised effectiveness of antidepressants with regard to the initial severity of depression: "Meta-analyses of antidepressant medications have reported only modest benefits over placebo treatment, and when unpublished trial data are included the benefit falls below accepted criteria for clinical significance antidepressant effectiveness." The conclusion the meta-analysis reached is that:

> Drug–placebo differences in antidepressant efficacy increase as a function of baseline severity, but are relatively small even for severely depressed patients. The relationship between initial severity and antidepressant efficacy is attributable to decreased responsiveness to placebo among very severely depressed patients, rather than to increased responsiveness to medication.[141]

This damn placebo is up to its old tricks again, ruining the good name of SSRIs.

But why? Why do SSRIs under the light of certain meta-analysis fail to beat placebos? There is an underlying theory after all, supporting them, a smart theory, the theory of "chemical imbalance". SSRIs, Selective Serotonin Reuptake Inhibitors, prevent the neurotransmitter called serotonin that has been released into the synaptic gap from being retaken into the presynaptic neurons, creating an effect that is equivalent to increased serotonin levels. More serotonin, more happiness? It sounds clever, and would be ingenious if it could only be proved that decreased serotonin levels played a decisive or definite role in depression. As it has been already mentioned, they tried to pull a similar con in the "appetite suppressant" class of drugs, namely in the Fen-phen case. And both classes of drugs sound alike and equally vague: "appetite suppressants" and "antidepressants" both deal with serotonin levels. Why not? Both classes of drugs sound smart. The only problem is that a smart theory does not equal a competent theory. In fact Dr. David Healy paralleled the serotonin-depression theory to the masturbatory theory of insanity:

> Both have been depletion theories, both have survived in spite of the evidence, both contain an implicit message as to what people ought to do. In the case of these myths, the key question is whose interests are being served by a widespread promulgation of such views rather than how do we test this theory.[142]

In an excellent, vibrant essay that is radiating reason, logic and scientific deontology, Jeffrey Lacasse and Jonathan Leo discuss about a disconnect between the advertisement and scientific literature regarding SSRIs and depression:

> Contemporary neuroscience research has failed to confirm any serotonergic lesion in any mental disorder, and has in fact provided significant counterevidence to the explanation of a simple neurotransmitter deficiency. Modern neuroscience has instead shown that the brain is vastly complex and poorly understood. While neuroscience is a rapidly advancing field,

to propose that researchers can objectively identify a "chemical imbalance" at the molecular level is not compatible with the extant science. In fact, there is no scientifically established ideal "chemical balance" of serotonin, let alone an identifiable pathological imbalance. To equate the impressive recent achievements of neuroscience with support for the serotonin hypothesis is a mistake.

With direct proof of serotonin deficiency in any mental disorder lacking, the claimed efficacy of SSRIs is often cited as indirect support for the serotonin hypothesis. Yet, this *ex juvantibus* line of reasoning (i.e. reasoning "backwards" to make assumptions about disease *causation* based on the response of the disease to a *treatment*) is logically problematic—the fact that aspirin cures headaches does not prove that headaches are due to low levels of aspirin in the brain. Serotonin researchers from the US National Institute of Mental Health Laboratory of Clinical Science clearly state, "The demonstrated efficacy of selective serotonin reuptake inhibitors...cannot be used as primary evidence for serotonergic dysfunction in the pathophysiology of these disorders."

Reasoning backwards, from SSRI efficacy to presumed serotonin deficiency, is thus highly contested. The validity of this reasoning becomes even more unlikely when one considers recent studies that even call into question the very efficacy of the SSRIs. Irving Kirsch and colleagues, using the Freedom of Information Act, gained access to all clinical trials of antidepressants submitted to the Food and Drug Administration (FDA) by the pharmaceutical companies for medication approval. When the published and unpublished trials were pooled, the placebo duplicated about 80% of the antidepressant response; 57% of these pharmaceutical company-funded trials failed to show a statistically significant difference between antidepressant and inert placebo. A recent Cochrane review suggests that these results are inflated as compared to trials that use an active placebo. This modest efficacy and extremely high rate of placebo response are not seen in the treatment of well-studied imbalances such as insulin deficiency, and casts doubt on the serotonin hypothesis.

Also problematic for the serotonin hypothesis is the growing body of research comparing SSRIs to interventions that do not target serotonin specifically. For instance, a Cochrane systematic review found no major difference in efficacy between SSRIs and tricyclic antidepressants. In addition, in randomized controlled trials, bupropion and reboxetine were just as effective as the SSRIs in the treatment of depression, yet neither affects serotonin to any significant degree. St. John's Wort and placebo have outperformed SSRIs in recent randomized controlled trials. Exercise was found to be as effective as the SSRI sertraline in a randomized controlled trial...

...Although SSRIs are considered "antidepressants", they are FDA-approved treatments for eight separate psychiatric diagnoses, ranging from social anxiety disorder to obsessive-compulsive disorder to premenstrual dysphoric disorder. Some consumer advertisements (such as the Zoloft and Paxil websites) promote the serotonin hypothesis, not just for depression, but also for some of these other diagnostic categories. Thus, for the serotonin hypothesis to be correct as currently presented, serotonin regulation would need to be the cause (and remedy) of each of these disorders. This is improbable, and no one has yet proposed a cogent theory explaining how a singular putative neurochemical abnormality could result in so many wildly differing behavioral manifestations.

In short, there exists no rigorous corroboration of the serotonin theory, and a significant body of contradictory evidence...

...However, in addition to what these authors say about serotonin, it is also important to look at what is *not* said in the scientific literature. To our knowledge, there is not a single peer-reviewed article that can be accurately cited to directly support claims of serotonin deficiency in any mental disorder, while there are many articles that present counterevidence."[143]

SSRIs are FDA approved for 8 separate psychiatric conditions... Well, we are not dealing with a chemical agent but with a kind of psychiatric "panacea". Do they also get rid of "bad spirits" and demons? The magic bullet effect seems to be very strong in SSRIs.

Anti-SSRI critique has been steadily building up. Dr. Joanna Moncrieff reportedly acknowledged: "It is high time that it was stated clearly that the serotonin imbalance theory of depression is not supported by the scientific evidence or by expert opinion. Through misleading publicity the pharmaceutical industry has helped to ensure that most of the general public is unaware of this."[144]

So, we have an unproven serotonergic hypothesis, drugs that work slightly better than placebo, if any better at all, yet the industry behaves and part of the medical community acts as if the hypothesis was a fact and as if the drugs delivered, luring troubled persons into SSRI treatment. Why?

It is simplistic medicine, Pulp Medicine all over again. It is easier and more attractive to ignore the "...multifactorial nature of depression and anxiety, and the ambiguities inherent in psychiatric diagnosis and treatment..."[145] and stick to the magic bullet effect. And it does wonders for the drug sales. Lacasse and Leo describe that: "Research has demonstrated that class-wide SSRI advertising has expanded the size of the antidepressant market, and SSRIs are now among the best-selling drugs in medical practice."[146] So when it comes to SSRIs, someone could describe the current situation as a coup de tat against science and society supported by a systematic propaganda attempting to medicalize normal behavior. The gold rush accompanying "mental illness" is not accepted by all.

In a laconic and profound release, the British House of Commons Health Committee concluded that SSRIs have been "indiscriminately prescribed on a grand scale," partly due to "data secrecy and uncritical acceptance of drug company views." SSRIs marketing strategies have "worked to persuade too many professionals that they can prescribe [the drugs] with impunity" to treat "unhappiness [that] is part of the spectrum of human experience, not a medical condition."[147] Lord Warner expressed his sentiments about the tendency of over-medicalization:

> I have some concerns that sometimes we do, as a society, wish to put labels on things which are just part and parcel of the human condition... Particularly in the area of depression we did ask the National Institute for Clinical Excellence to look into this particular area and their guideline on depression did advise non-pharmacological treatment for mild depression.[148]

And it is not only about over simplistic approaches, bad science, greed and an unproductive public health extravaganza.

Dr. David Healy has for long now been exploring a possible relation between SSRIs and derivative suicidal thoughts on patients under SSRI treatment. The industry, of course, rebuffed Healy's claims as expected. Drug-related suicide does not only kill the suicidal. It damages antidepressant sales as well. In October 2004, the FDA, under the light of a study that vindicated Healy's thesis for SSRI-induced suicide, ordered black box warnings on SSRI labels informing of an increased suicide risk.

We are all biological machines. We are also social and mental entities. We are also preservers and promoters of knowledge, treasurers of emotions and memories, catalysts of change and, last but not least, we are Living. To be a living organism, a complicated, sentient, living organism is an experience that cannot be fragmented into tiny pieces of information. Life sciences have to immediately reevaluate their perspective and embrace life as a whole.

Psychiatry and the man-machine model has failed woefully. It is unable to keep up with the requirements and needs of modern living. It has articulated laughable theories, reprehensible practices and pathetic excuses. The "science" that is supposed to understand the human adventure better than any other discipline behaves as if it was studying extraterrestrial oddities.

Any human being has the right to refuse any treatment that will diminish it, or perceive it or handle it as a broken machine or as a piece of meat. We are that, definitely so, but we are also more, much more. Life sciences are constantly disregarding the higher aspects of the human entity, constantly humiliating and assaulting each and every one of us.

And we do have alternatives. And the alternatives definitely look better, and probably work better as well. Exercise has been found to relieve patients from the symptoms of depression.[149] Furthermore, continued exercise has been shown to prevent depression relapses. A study in 2000, comparing exercise to medication, concluded that only 8% of patients in the exercise group had their depression return, while 38% of the drug-only group and 31% of the exercise-plus-drug group relapsed. One of the leading researchers provided an interpretation for this disproportionate response to treatment:

Simply taking a pill is very passive... Patients who exercised may have felt a greater sense of mastery over their condition and gained a greater sense of accomplishment. They may have felt more self-confident and competent because they were able to do it themselves, and attributed their improvement to their ability to exercise. Once patients start feeling better, they tend to exercise more, which makes them feel even better, Blumenthal said.[150]

But instead of motivating patients and encouraging self-empowerment, psychiatrists choose to turn them into blind instruments of drug consumption and addiction. And this approach is rather disastrous.

Mosher commented on the plight and the future of psychiatry:

> We are all just helplessly caught up in a swirl of brain pathology for which no one, except DNA, is responsible...
>
> I view with no surprise that psychiatric training is being systematically disavowed by American medical school graduates. This must give us cause for concern about the state of today's psychiatry. It must mean – at least in part that they view psychiatry as being very limited and unchallenging. To me it seems clear that we are headed toward a situation in which, except for academics, most psychiatric practitioners will have no real relationships – so vital to the healing process – with the disturbed and disturbing persons they treat. Their sole role will be that of prescription writers – ciphers in the guise of being "helpers".[151]

We have created an inhuman drug pushing culture, a culture that is adopting, encouraging and regulated by uppers, downers and fixers. We are engaged in an extensive drug dealing enterprise, yet we advice our boys and girls to keep away from street drugs. Do you thing we sound convincing?

*c) Why doctors will give you only half-truths about...*
**Expanding Psychiatric Definitions onto the Healthy and Unsuspecting**
DSM was originally 130 pages long, listing 106 mental disorders.

Gradually it expanded. The ever-inflating DSM in its current edition lists 297 disorders in 886 pages. Have people become more colorfully insane over time? Perhaps. Have the psychiatric pseudosciences become more precise and knowledgeable? Could be so. Or is it that there is an expansive policy, a psychiatric imperialism that is trying to colonize and control healthy populations? Definitely so. Psychiatric definitions are voraciously expanding and if this tendency is left unchecked and uncontrolled it could engulf pretty much all of us.

In the 18th and early 19th centuries, psychiatry targeted among others the "feeble-minded". I never actually understood what this kind of elusive definition, as elusive as bad blood or ether, actually implied or described, and I bet that none of its contemporary shrinks understood it either. So they had the freedom and luxury to pretty much turn it against anyone who wasn't strong enough or important enough to defend himself against it.

The pseudoscientific DSM used to incorporate gay people. Homosexuality used to be a disorder. It was not until gay activists did what they had to do, that it is, act against it, that the DSM priesthood was forced to remove homosexuality from their "hit list", their grocery shopping list.

And this is called science? No, this is no science. This is politics. Loren Mosher pointed out that the DSM and psychiatry today have become "… a matter of fashion, politics and, like the pharmaceutical house connection, money."

And Mosher did more then to just simply sketch out the problem. He wielded a fierce and profound critique on his profession, his guild and its dominant mindset:

Finally, why must the APA pretend to know more than it does? DSM IV is the fabrication upon which psychiatry seeks acceptance by medicine in general. Insiders know it is more a political than scientific document. To its credit it says so – although its brief apologia is rarely noted. DSM IV has

160

become a bible and a money-making best-seller – its major failings notwithstanding. It confines and defines practice, some take it seriously, others more realistically. It is the way to get paid. Diagnostic reliability is easy to attain for research projects. The issue is what do the categories tell us? Do they in fact accurately represent the person with a problem? They don't, and can't, because there are no external validating criteria for psychiatric diagnoses. There is neither a blood test nor specific anatomic lesions for any major psychiatric disorder. So, where are we? APA as an organization has implicitly (sometimes explicitly as well) bought into a theoretical hoax. Is psychiatry a hoax – as practiced today? Unfortunately, the answer is mostly yes.[152]

This hoax was finally understood by the gay activists that managed to free homosexual preference from the DSM canonistic claws. The DSM, under social evolutional pressure, had to evolve itself. But towards what direction? As Louise Armstrong noted, "To read about the evolution of the DSM is to know this: it is an entirely political document. What it includes, what it does not include, are the result of intensive campaigning, lengthy negotiating, infighting, and power plays."[153]

Having lost such a huge clientele, the DSM priesthood had to replenish their lost resources and influence with something new, something fresh. Fish out a new target group.

If DSM is a political manifesto at its very core, then why shouldn't it turn to politics to expand even further?

Well I was a bit surprised to find out that it already did. Geoffrey D. White came up with an exciting new product: Political Apathy Disorder[154] which according to the Huffington Post is under consideration for the upcoming DSM V.[155] I was flabbergasted, stunned, rendered speechless. At first I thought it was a prank, a joke like the one the brilliant Ray Moynihan pulled on us with his hilarious MDD (motivational deficiency disorder), a psychiatric approach to laziness, showing us how easily pretty much anything could be medicalized.[156] If it wasn't a joke, well then the joke is on us. And if the joke is incorporated into DSM V, well it is not funny anymore. It is a direct threat to democracy. Approximately 70% of the human species, the politically apathetic version of it, will be under psychiatry's jurisdiction.

Let's look at the diagnostic criteria of this disorder. The perfect PAD:

1. Spends at least twice as much money on vacations as on alleviating social problems (poverty, health care, racism, education, corporate welfare, campaign finance issues etc.).

2. Owns an SUV (sports utility vehicle). These are dirty (four times more toxic emissions than regular cars) and dangerous (10 times greater mortality rate for non-SUVs that collide with them.

3. Owns a minivan, which has three to five times the emissions of a regular vehicle.

4. Invests in non-SRI (socially responsible investing) mutual funds, pension plans, 401k etc. If an individual (or the company for which he works) has non-SRI investments, there are no prohibitions against investing in tobacco stocks, weapons industry, alcoholic beverage companies etc.

5. Buys Starbucks Coffee. This company is now owned by Philip Morris (the world's largest tobacco company). Further, Starbucks exploits small Third World coffee growers and has contributed to a feudal-like system in these countries.

6. Purchases any of the following products, which are owned by Philip Morris: Grape-Nuts, Miller beer, Miracle Whip, Sanka, Post cereals, Kraft Macaroni and Cheese,

Minute Rice, Shake 'n Bake, Shreddies, Cool Whip, Cracker Barrel cheeses, Maxwell House coffee, Philadelphia Cream Cheese, and Cheez Whiz.

7. Lives in a gated community.
8. Verbalizes concern about social problems and human suffering but does nothing about them, i.e. confuses moral sentiment with moral action.
9. Believes that morality is completely defined by merely avoiding harm to others (has never considered that morality means helping those in need when possible).
10. Knows more names for coffee drinks (latte, cappuccino, espresso) than names of members of the Cabinet.
11. Believes that freedom of speech is more important than "one person/ one vote".
12. Doesn't read the ballot pamphlet until in the voting booth.
13. Is opposed to social welfare but not corporate welfare, even though more is spent on the latter.
14. Believes that the federal government should spend more on the defense budget than on social programs.
15. Failed to vote in two or more (local, state, national) elections in the last two years.
16. Has spent more time remodeling their home than on involvement in a political campaign or project.
17. Buys shoes and sports equipment (especially made by Nike) manufactured by child and sweatshop labor typically in Third World countries.

I still wonder if anyone wrote this seriously and I am still very hesitant to copy this (I am still afraid that Ray Moynihan has played another educating prank under a pseudonym this time). OK, White got it all right about political apathy, and this description would make perfect sense if it wasn't for one thing: this indifference towards others is not a psychiatric phenomenon, it is a cultural and socio-political one. Some thousand years ago, the Ancient Greeks described the same phenomenon. They used a particularly strong word for it: the word idiocy. Idiot meant private individual and idiocy meant privacy, in the sense of unwillingness or disinterest to participate in public matters. Now, they knew they had to live with this, they didn't condone it but there was not much more they could do than educate, motivate and inspire people. They didn't make drink offerings to the Olympian Gods to treat their city for idiocy nor did they resort to the oracle's advice to treat the condition.

The author describes this idiocy in psychiatric terms and no matter how well-intentioned one is another one might always wonder: does it take one to know one?

The politically apathetic disturbed (PADs) people are a vast majority on this planet and it is very unlikely that they'll be targeted by the DSMV. This is a great opportunity though for DSM to finally turn out helpful and promote a therapeutic cause, because, if the psychopriesthood decides to incorporate the PADs in DSMV, there is a good chance they'll be miraculously cured of their apathy, turn political and turn against DSMV and psychiatry. No, that's too risky. Let's stick to what DSM knows best. Attack and engulf minorities, vulnerable and, even better, defenseless minorities.

Well, judging from the declining interest of the modern world in parenting, kids, yes, why not, kids would be just perfect. Perfect mental patients. Why not? They seem defenseless enough.

And it has been done before. Pseudoscience favors segregation, authoritarianism and the total disregard of dignity, free will, individuality and civil rights.

As Fuller Torrey described:

DSM-IV, published in 1994, includes as mental disorders such behaviors as "disorder of written expression", "childhood conduct disorder", "pathological gambling", "adjustment disorder with anxiety", and "avoidant personality disorder". The boundaries of such "disorders" are so vague that I can find a DSM-IV diagnosis to fit everyone I know – except of course my wife.

It was precisely this mishmash of vague psychiatric categories that in the 1980s enabled the Psychiatric Institutes of America (PIA) and National Medical Enterprises Inc. (recently reborn as Tenet Healthcare Corp) to imprison adolescent children in private psychiatric hospitals until their insurance ran out (brilliantly chronicled by Joe Sharkey in Bedlam).[157]

Joe Sharkey's *Bedlam* describes incidents that traumatized humanity. It is a story of what happens when greed meets pseudoscience, prejudice and social indifference.[158]

Children are targeted and brutally hurt or even emotionally disabled. It has happened before, during the late 18th and the early 19th centuries under the vague definition of "feeble-mindedness". It happened again in the 1980s. And it is happening again under DSM IV.

### d) Why doctors will give you only half-truths about...
### ADHD – A Disease in the Definition

"Fetch," I enthusiastically shouted but to no avail.

The ball passed by a disinterested dog and landed to the grass some yards away from him, unchallenged, unclaimed.

OK, I was the one who was doing the fetching. Again.

I kneeled and patted the dog softly on his head.

"What's wrong with you, boy? Why can't you be just like all other normal dogs and go fetch a ball? Is that too much to ask for a dog?"

The dog looked meaningfully at the far side of the park and off he was to his favorite butterfly chasing.

This dog is never going to make anything great out of himself.

He should become a poet but dogs don't get to become poets, I thought sorrowfully, but kept the thoughts to myself not to hurt his feelings.

But I wasn't the only one with problems or the only one who was keeping thoughts to himself not to hurt other people's feelings. At the direction that the dog was facing a moment ago there was a father standing, throwing a softball at his son, waiting for him to strike it with his clumsily-held baseball bat.

But the boy was clearly not interested in baseball. He appeared to be interested in everything else, the grass, the dog, the butterflies, me, but not the ball. The ball landed on the grass, some yards from the boy, unchallenged, unclaimed.

It was as if I could hear the father's disappointment resounding in my head: Why can't you just be like all other normal boys and hit a ball? Is that too much to ask for a boy?

Then it struck me, almost as hard as a baseball bat: the dog and the boy were co-patients. I mean I may not be a psychiatrist, but it was crystal clear even to the eyes of the untrained, wasn't it? The boy and the dog shared the same medical condition: ADHD, Attention Deficit Hyperactive Disorder.

Four letter medical abbreviations were almost a perfect match for three letter words like boy or kid and, hey, why not a dog?

I was thrilled with my finding. I had killed with the ADHD diagnosis two birds, well not two birds but rather a boy and a dog.

I dashed home to go refresh my DSM, the Statistical Manual of Mental Disorders, currently in its fourth edition. I opened the psychiatric bible, the great book that defines and separates the good from the damaged, the ordinary people from the deranged, the normal fellows from the nutcases, the functional from the certifiable, the people who are allowed a certain degree of exercising their free will from the cuckoos that need to be checked, supervised, restrained or regulated.

There it was: instant enlightenment. According to DSMIV,

ADHD is defined as a:

> persistent pattern of inattention or hyperactivity—impulsivity that is more frequently displayed and more severe than is typically observed in individuals at a comparable level of development.

In science it is critical for definitions to define the conditions or terms they attempt to define as thoroughly as possible.

So what is it then? Inattention or hyperactivity? Both? A bit of the one and a bit of the other? A racemic mixture of them? It is obvious that the two terms are not identical, and more often than not seem to even contradict each other. Hyperactivity does require attention in the very thing they want to be active in, with a corresponding disinterest in the thing you want them to be interested in. Normal people who are not interested in something will naturally find their attention shift away. If it shifts away quickly, is that a disorder? Do people who lose interest quickly, with their attention also shifting away quickly to something else, really have a disorder or a disorder related to being impulsive? Yet the same kids can run around and play games that they like.

And so let's look at it again: *"...impulsivity that is more frequently displayed and more severe than is typically observed..."*

More frequently displayed... Meaning? How often, I mean like every ten seconds, every minute, every hour? And what about *"severe impulsivity"*? What does severe impulsivity mean? To be honest I have never heard a human creature accusing another as being severely impulsive. Too impulsive for his own good perhaps, but severely impulsive? And what is the golden standard to which ADHD persons are compared to? But of course the typically observed impulsivity. The typically observed impulsivity. It has a nice ring to it as if it was meaning or describing or actually defining anything. What behavior is typical? Or perhaps the definition refers to typical observers, or to typical acceptance amongst typical experts on what constitutes typical behavior? Where do they come up with such ill-defined definitions of illness?

And that brings us to critically look at what is to be typical. Was Einstein typical? Was Newton typical? Was Leonardo da Vinci typical? Was Galileo typical? And do you want to be typical? An impulsive response may not be typical but is it always part of a disorder? And what disorderly biochemistry typifies it?

A typical impulsivity in Harvard Law School is not the same as the typical impulsivity in the streets of Harlem. The typical modern behavior has nothing to do with the typical Victorian behavior. Things that are considered scandalous or way out of limits in one place today were considered as normal, accepted, well tolerated and even expected in other societies of the past and the present and vice versa.

Typical equals dictatorial. *Typical* and normal is a powerful instrument that authorities and societies use to elicit and impose accepted and, desirable for them, behaviors and marginalize problematic (for them) behaviors and isolate possible and actual troublemakers. But it is the law's task to deal with troublemakers, not psychiatry's. Psychiatry has to deal with troubled people and that should be enough of a task to keep her occupied.

Typical has nothing to do with mental health. Nevertheless, it has everything to do with social, political and scientific conformism. And what exactly is the definition of mental health except from the opposite of not being normal, sane and *typical*? We are missing something crucial here, something crucial and evident. We are missing a complete definition of mental health. Without it we are doomed to fall prey to misconceptions, distortions and public mental health abuses.

Loose definitions, ill-defined terms, populist rhetorics. There you have it: a recipe for a successful psychiatric disorder. And if disorderly biochemistry typifies the particular definition, does it call for treatment with drugs as drugs are not typically found in the typically "normal" people or do you go back to proper food and clinical nutrition to address the biochemistry in the brain? I mean, what would then constitute a typically appropriate treatment, if one should avoid being impulsive about using drugs. The logic, if it does draw any serious and lasting attention, revolves around the fact that drugs can alter the normal biochemistry in the brain, in the first place. Naturally the question that pops up is, so why this impulsive rush to introduce such toxic chemicals into the central nervous system of which the brain is a part?

It would be of less significance if the issue was only scientific or if the issue was brought up only for the sake of argument. It is not about creating an argument for its own sake but rather to find a meaningful basis to look at the definitions that in themselves create problematic situations. On the other hand, if there is a health problem, at all, relating to an observed non-typical behavior involving attention or hyperactivity, it must be scientifically defined with some reference to an underlying cause, whether biochemical and other factors such that it also affords clear and proper categorization rather than conflict it by wrapping it up in contradictory possibilities, before classifying it as a disorder.

Without the support of underlying cause factors it appears not only superficial but also contorted and these types of definitions appear more as part of a make-believe instead of biochemical or causative science for what may be observed as atypical must be accompanied by some changes in biochemistry or pathology or infection etc etc. Unfortunately, the field of psychiatry does not take that direction.

About 3–4% of the general population is diagnosed with ADHD. Unfortunately children are especially targeted by this make-believe disorder. Some of them are medicated to treat their condition. And with what may I ask? With methylphenidate, an amphetamine derivative.

Here is an illegal substance that poses serious personal and social hazards when it is sold on the streets but we wisely choose to prescribe and use it to treat our children from an ill-defined illness at best, an imaginary disease at worse so we can wash our hands from the labors and hardships of raising a child or teaching a child. With every single step we take towards this direction, the direction of handing more and more of our power and responsibilities to authorities, the more weak and disempowered we become. And it is not as if the experts know exactly what they are doing. Behavior and emotion are outcomes and expressions of a vast biochemical universe whose laws and regulatory mechanisms, to be perfectly honest, we don't exactly know. It is a complex web of biochemical pathways some of which like the hormones are not within the central nervous system. The natural antioxidant system plays an important part and the redox balance can impact or alter these biochemical pathways resulting in change in thinking patterns and behavioral changes, and culture itself is a major conditioning factor of such behavior and thinking patterns and responses. The bottom line issue is the complexity of healthy biochemistry. So, we are jumping towards judging the book by the cover, the entire "innerverse" by certain behaviors we don't approve and intervening at specific biochemical spots to disrupt certain patterns of behavior. It is the same shallow medical approach all over again: As long as you treat the symptom who cares about the cause?

Even if we knew, even if we knew exactly in biochemical terms what conditions generate specific "unwanted" behaviors, would we be ready to give up individuality for the sake of a neatly arrayed, uniform, chemically or genetically regulated behavior? Are we ready to transform into a Hive society?

And why try only amphetamines? Shouldn't we also try cocaine on children and turn them into state and psychiatry controlled junkies so they can cope better in school and in home? Shouldn't we as a society discuss about substance use or abuse before they are imposed to us under a scientific garment? Or should we make scientific attempts to shift away from drug-controlled and drug-modified behaviors and attention spans?

If only we knew what generates behavior and desires. If only we knew the exact underlying biochemical mechanisms responsible for ADHD wouldn't that be absolutely great?

But who said the cause of ADHD is biochemical?

Boring…

Boring…

You can hear children repeating this word over and over again.

Whose fault is it that kids get bored at school? Or if something will not be presented to them in ways that they find interesting or in ways that elicits some form of interaction from their developing neocortex? Maybe what is felt as desirable and interesting to the adult ends up in the crocodilian processes and appears as intensely boring. Many children do not like repetitive tasks that they find boring but adults find interesting and give due attention to it.

Booooring…

Who is responsible for not turning the learning experience into an attractive and interesting process?

Albert Einstein is a historic figure who gave intense attention to non-typical things and would probably fit into the ADHD diagnostic criteria if they existed in his time. Albert as a child was an underachiever and his teachers complained about him not paying any attention to them. Probably he was not interested in the typical and repetitive things that they did in class. Who could possibly blame little Albert; I mean the kid had a different and more interesting universe waiting to be discovered in his head and the urge was pressing – much bigger and something more dynamic. Why should he devote his intellect to conformist teachers teaching 18<sup>th</sup> and 19<sup>th</sup> centuries' gospel as if it was god's words and laws: eternal, everlasting, inescapable, and undeviating? If we had ADHD and pumped young Albert with Ritalin back then, presumably Albert would be better focused and have gotten better grades, his parents and his teachers would be happy about his improvement but presumably we would have restricted his daydreaming, his pondering, his ability to drift in and out of the intellectual ether. Presumably, to "cure" one person and make a few others happier for a while, we could have set back physics for a decade, a century or even more.

A discovery-oriented mind is not a typical mind. Such a mind cannot focus on repetitive tasks. It quickly gets bored with repetition. It needs to do more things and move on in its quest to find joy and fun in discovery voyages of its own or in participation. If it cannot drive in discovery it will not give attention. So, unless there are proper and certain underlying causative factors such as redox imbalances or biochemical changes with or without inflammatory changes or such disturbances associated with heavy metals from perfumes or some other source, one should look at the picture again. What about chemicals and drugs and painkillers used or consumed during pregnancy? Try to get a more complete picture. Probe scientifically.

I remembered the kid with the baseball bat. What if he was a new Einstein forced by his father to get interested in baseball or by his mother to take his Ritalin?

Then I remembered of something else that had to do with Ritalin, ADHD or ADD and, awkwardly, baseball.

During the George Mitchell probe into Major League Baseball steroid abuse when MLB records where handed over to congressional investigators, a very interesting finding surfaced. The number of athletes that were taking Ritalin, Adderall and other drugs to deal with their "Attention Deficit Disorder" skyrocketed from 28 to 103 within one year. A total of 7.8% of MLB athletes were all of a sudden diagnosed with ADD and were permitted to have "therapeutic use exemptions" from baseball's ampheta-mines ban.[159]

There is every reason to believe that this fivefold increase in MLB ADD diagnosis did not occur because of underlying medical conditions but rather because some of the super athletes and their doctors, so accustomed to the amphetamine fix, found a way to circumvent the ban and get the extra benefits of the performance-enhancer drugs.

There is no doubt about it. The danger in drugs is that while they can induce secretions or quickly induce the production of biochemicals like dopamine from brain tissue, their metabolism in mammalian cells yields large amounts of hydrogen peroxide which must be quickly converted into water and oxygen by the SOD-glutathione-catalase enzyme system. Over time, drug use can lead to depletion of these enzymes and minerals such as zinc, copper, iron and manganese that catalytically enhance its role. The steady depletion of enzymes and minerals in the brain cells can lead to excess free radicals or excess hydrogen peroxide. Excess free radicals can establish inflammatory changes in brain cells while excess hydrogen peroxide can alter the biochemical pathways. During this process there could be vitamin B depletion as well and sufficient depletion will certainly impair the healthy functioning of nervous tissue and interfere with the healthy functioning of the neocortex and the pineal gland. Sleep quality could deteriorate and the amount of human growth hormone and melatonin produced at night during sleep could decrease, especially in a state of excess free radical and mineral deficiency. And as the healthy biochemistry gets altered it can affect output as well as thinking. Mild headaches can become more frequent. Drugs will never be the answer to correcting redox imbalances and natural antioxidant and organic mineral deficiencies. Those answers lie in clinical nutrition and food. Unfortunately, modern society treats kids with performance enhancer drugs because we don't like we the way they act or

Pulp Med

don't act, turning normal kids into psychiatric patients as we take on the grand role of glorified drug pushers just because it was so hard to raise a kid or to get his attention.

And as you begin to probe more scientifically and begin to step away from the psychiatric and pharmaceutical virtuality you open your vision to a wide range of alternative solutions out there. First and foremost is love and understanding and the power to generate a spark of interest in the kid's mind and soul, to encourage it to find exactly that in which it will excel. And there are other solutions too

Dr. John J. Ratey, an associate professor of psychiatry at Harvard Medical School and the author of "Spark: The Revolutionary New Science of Exercise and the Brain" described to Newsweek that: "The intense physical activity fosters a level of focus and commitment that helps the athlete improve the functioning of the brain. In fact, athletic competition can be the best cure for ADD,"[160] but always support athletic activity with nutrition based on fresh fruit and vegetables for the natural antioxidants and minerals, not forgetting the medium-chain fatty acids and small amounts of oils that have fat-soluble antioxidants. If you take supplements make sure that they are not synthetic but natural and formulated from edible plants and herbs that are rich in antioxidants and minerals.

Intense mental activity would be an excellent exercise as well. And what a great idea it would be if we played Mozart's music in school classes, which has been proven to augment spatial reasoning skills.[161]

Yes there are a lot of alternative reliable approaches out there. But we choose almost entirely to rely upon the "magic pill effect". It is effortless, demands nothing of us, so why not use it?

Come to think of it, it be would so convenient for myself and thousands of other authors if the writer's block and the prior-to-writing stress were to be cleverly defined as mental disorders and we either had free access to performance-enhancing drugs like

Ritalin or be forced to take them. Pharmaceutically-induced inspiration, wit, and clarity, what more can a writer ask for? There is a heavy price though to be paid when a simple problem of disinterest or quick shifts in attention develop into real problems in brain biochemistry induced by drug use: addiction, familiarization of the receptors and sometimes serious side effects like suicidal thoughts and personality alterations.

Yes, you are probably right. These drugs are too dangerous for writers. Let's stick to the recipe and give medicalized "speed" only to children.

### e) Why doctors will give you only half-truths about...
### ODD, the Oddest Disorder of Them All

Gill is a little devil. She is giving her teachers in school a hard time; her mother describes the hardships of bringing her up as a living hell. The odd thing about Gill is that apart from her irritating, nerve-breaking behavior, besides her fighting temper, her constant fallouts with other children, she is an excellent student and a first-class athlete, a striking contrast that makes her parents even more uncomfortable and embarrassed. The kid is a first-class material, her teachers think, her problems must originate from her upbringing. But her parents have done nothing to upset or trigger such a behavior in Gill. In fact, her parents are peace-loving persons, never got in trouble with the law or their neighbors, they are successful professionals, in other words role models for the local community.

The family's emotional balance is torn apart. Not a moment of peace, not a single word uttered to the child that won't be argued, not a single exhortation unchallenged, not a nudge without an outburst, let alone commands. Everything is questioned, challenged, disobeyed. Sometimes her parents ask themselves who is really the parent and who is the child in this relationship, who has the upper hand, who is in control. Because the pair most certainly is not. In fact the whole situation appears to be totally out of control, completely unmanageable. And who can blame the poor parents? They are doing their best in bringing up a teenage Hulk. It is only natural that most of the time they find themselves at a loss. There was nothing left for them to do except to seek for help, the kind of help that only experts can offer. But besides their declared intention for professional help, they didn't even know where to turn to until they read about ODD: Oppositional Defiant Disorder. The parents were relieved that Gill was an ODD child, a psychiatric patient and not a unique unexplained phenomenon of childhood disobedience and irritability. 5 to 15% of all children exhibit this disorder. After the expert treatment, Gill was a different child, a tolerable child. She lost her appetite for fight and alongside she lost a little piece of her aptness to learning and her proneness in sportsmanship but that was a small price to pay. Gill didn't feel alone anymore, didn't feel different or special and felt like she had nothing to defend for or to defend against. The psychiatric intervention had performed miracles with Gill and turned her into somewhat of a normal child. The war of the soul was over; the family could at last leave in peace, unhindered by Gill's outbursts.

Kevin was much more of a troublemaker than Gill could ever hope to be. When he was a child he set his sister's tree house on fire. Unfortunately for Kevin and the other 5 to 15% of the children of his era there was no ODD diagnosis at the time. In contrast with Gill, Kevin went on with his problematic life and continued having troubles. He was kicked out of Northridge Military Academy for throwing a tire at a fellow student. It was obvious that the boy and juvenile Kevin was nothing but a troublemaker and that he would go on with his life aimlessly, wasting his time over quarrels and making others lose their temper, a rebel without a cause. It was not until Kevin discovered that he could take his extra energy and his defiance into acting, into the art that extends and at sometimes defies the private personality, that Kevin would materialize his ODD into full-blown self-expression and he would learn to turn a problem and disadvantage into a productive virtue that would render him lovable, earn him respect from his peers along with two Oscars. The problematic tornado-boy was none other than Kevin Spacey.

And one cannot help but wonder: if a psycho expert had gotten hold of the defiant oppositional Kevin-child, and smoothed it a little bit at the edges, who would Kevin be today? A self-sufficient pastry-maker? An acknowledged military man? Kevin could as well be in someone else's shoes just because his surroundings couldn't bear with him anymore and would have no option other than to hand him over to the psychiatric tan yard.

Five to fifteen percent of children today are suffering from this disorder. Amongst them are Gills and Kevins and other unique persons that will produce and extend their name, fame and work beyond their small original social environments, children that will gradually transform their anger and unconformity into a mature and true-blue form of expression, ugly ducklings that may evolve personally to became contributors to current and future civilizations. Nature has a tendency to promote diversities that may appear useless and annoying but serve her well, even protect her against a multitude of unpredicted future scenarios. Societies are no exception. But let's take a closer look at the diagnostic criteria of this widespread paidopsychiatric disorder. An ODD child's improper conduct is consisting of:

1. frequent outbursts
2. excessive arguing with adults
3. active defiance and refusal to comply with adult requests and rules
4. deliberate attempts to annoy or upset people
5. blaming others for his or her mistakes or misbehavior
6. often being touchy or easily annoyed by others

7. frequent anger and resentment
8. mean and hateful talking when upset
9. seeking revenge

But these symptoms all are part of childhood mental vigor aren't they? Being captious might make other people sick but that doesn't mean that being captious equals being sick. The only children that are not partly ODD are deceased ones. The alive ones, as far as I can remember, have feelings, real feelings that adults seem to often forget, blindly following the endless must-haves, must-dos of everyday life. But the kid, ah the kid is a multiuse tool of evolution, society's, spirit's, mind's and soul's evolution, a kid is pure potential. It is so normal for a kid to question, to argue, to challenge what is projected to it, or expected of it; it is so normal for a kid to try to dismantle the icy fixed world of musts and dos around it. This is the normal social experimentation root for kids. To challenge the norm, to see how far they can stretch it and get away with it. Children are by definition revolutionary and thus evolutionary.

But mental health experts wish behavior to be supervised, checked. Where there is an issue of control there is eagerness to interfere. I bet Big Brother hired mental health experts first to exercise complete power and control. Definitions are deliberately extended, sickness and disorder elbow out health and normality; it is a battlefield out there and children will not be spared.

OK, every child more or less exhibits ODD behaviors, the experts give us that much. But when is a child really ODD? Well, most symptoms must be repeated at least 2 or 3 times a week. Two to three times a week? Wow, that's a record high. No wonder that ODD estimates put the overall ODD incidence at a 5-15 percentage. ODD loves children to the point of pedophilia.

There is no doubt that there are some well-intentioned parents out there who are having a hard time with their "odd" children. Out of respect for them, we ought to consider that there are some extreme "odd" cases that the parent is incapable of handling by himself. Granted, psychiatry is mostly an art of the extremities, when behaviors of the normal specter are quantified in such a density and intensity that are incompatible with social life. Granted. Psychiatry categorizes and lists the extremities in behavior, and every behavior can reach extremities. So it is only natural to expect that extreme obedience and extreme compliance to be equally "psychiatrized" and represented in the psychiatric Mosaic Law of the DSM IV (Diagnostic and Statistical Manual of Mental Disorders). But then again, there is no such type of disorder in the DSM. And the reason for this absence is that such a behavioral extremity does not upset societies. No one will ever complain about a submissive child, no one will sent it to a psychiatrist even of it totally lacks essential qualities for character development such as courage, curiosity and imagi-nation. Submissive, obedient kids are dream children for their parents; they make convenient mates, disciplined soldiers, faithful flocks, converging costumers, manipulated voters. They are the backbone of society. No matter that there is always a good chance that this uniform child will never become self-fulfilled, never become a real person but only a shadow of imposed musts and shoulds, a spirit of Christmas past, an indistinguishable link on the long chain of traditionalism and conservatism, a ghost image of things handed down, a breakwater of change, the great and mediocre anti-catalyst for innovation; never, ever will he rise up above the underlying social matrix and become a civilization contributor such as Kevin and thousands of other acknowledged personalities. That is OK with societies and their psychiatry. It is fine with me also. Not anyone is supposed to excel, to differ, or divert from the mainstream and create his very own path, societies need elements of stability to remain coherent. Just as long as we don't demonize the opposite behavior and hunt down the ODD persons, people who just don't fit in prefab slots of the social matrix and strive to create their own discreet social signature. The steppenwolfs are a species in danger; they should be protected and not killed under the pretext that they endanger the flocks.

Talking of steppenwolfs, the author of Der Steppenwolf, the Nobelist Hermann Hesse was clearly an odd case, another boy that achieved greatness through his oddity. In continuous contrast with his surroundings, boy-Hermann was struggling to escape from his conservative upbringings and retain his personal color, his very own tune of thought, his uniqueness. Sent from one institute to another, committed even to a mental institute during his childhood to cope with his rebelliousness, Hermann survived with huge scars to create milestone literature for the whole of the Western civilization. It is fortunate that they didn't have ODD back then: while a scientifically-grounded psychiatric intervention could have made Hermann's parents lives happier and even boy-Hermann's life more tolerable, our civilization would have never received Hermann's meaningful agonies and ordeals, his bitter fruits of passion.

Judging from Hermann's case, one cannot help but wonder. Is there something wrong, psychiatrically wrong with the 5-15% of children nowadays or perhaps the problem lies in the very own societies that nurture them? Because the conflict between the odd children and their surroundings should not de facto be deemed as causeless or irrational. In Hermann's case, he grew up in a conservative environment consisting of rigid, non-productive schemes of thinking, and hypocritical behaviors dominated by religious behests. Being ODD was Hermann's best self-defense against an environment that sought to alter his soul, his idiosyncrasy, his mental capacity, his very own nature and turn him into a useful and acceptable social apparatus.

So if we are to diagnose a single case of the ODD child, we have to re-evaluate our Western civilization values, we have to look deeply into the social essence and its circumstances and ask ourselves a very hard question: in the settings that we have created for the children in the 21st century society, does a child have a reason to be ODD, is ODD intuitively-driven frustration and anger towards life and living in the 21st century? Is ODD not an reflection of an upward trend in childhood disorders, but rather a marker for the advent of conservatism, uniformity, homogenization and a meter of social intolerance towards difference?

Think of Hermann and Kevin, struggling against society's intolerance. Now imagine that they have also have to face a materialized figure of authority, a psychiatrist, telling them, pushing them, fingering for their Achilles heel, seeking for an entry point in their world of childhood resistance and persistence. The odd child has no word on his own future. It cannot complain because being a certified ODD child his complaints are de facto without good reason, mere symptoms of his disorder. The ODD child has to comply to the psychiatrist's instructions otherwise his syndromes will be viewed as persistent, his disorder will be deemed regressive, and he will be mercilessly treated until he becomes obsessive, an obsessive yes-Mr.-Dad, yes-Mr.-Dr., yes-Mr.-Teacher child. No way out for the ODD child. The treatment is a pincer movement, an iron maiden. And the first step towards "treatment", as in most psychiatric approaches, is to admit that they have a problem, to admit that they are simply ODD, not Kevins and Hermanns, simply ODD, and to declare their intention to be treated. Pretty much like the witch trials, where ignorant people had to confess first and repent afterwards. Either way, they were burned to the stake. It's a witch hunt all over again. Witch hunting is conservatism's fox hunt, a deadly sport related to social class. Gay people know only too well of the habit. They were hunted, and they had a good taste of what it feels like to be included in the DSM religious texts. Gayism is no longer a disorder; this is definitely good news, people fought, and fought hard to earn the right be viewed as normal, but instead, angry childhood is? There can be no angry children's union, no social pressure exercised by a unanimous accordance of repressed children, no minority request. No, children are easy prey, little foxes killed for fun, a novel minority that the psychiatric priesthood decided to define just for the kicks of it. And children are helpless against this authoritarian minority, as helpless as a child can be. And now that the ODD child was been irritated inside of me, I feel like passing some expert advice to the experts counselors, free of charge: Well, noble psychiatrist and ODD expert, really, get a real job or pick up a fight against someone your own size.

The malice of the ODD segmentation does not stop with destroying the potential for greatness of oddly beautiful and oddly different children. OK we are supposed to live in an era of prosperity and peace. ODD one could argue is useless in our times. But if ODD is eliminated or "treated", I wonder, when things turn bad, who will pick up a fight against a bad teacher, or a molester, or a soul strangler, or a tyrant of nations, a wrongdoer of any kind? Will it be the submissive compliant child, or the submissive, compliant, socially-acceptable adult? Do not think so. It is the ODD reservoir that will provide society with righteous revolutionaries. Nature creates behavioral molecules that will be activated when the time is right, and it is creating them in abundance so it may never run out of them in times of need. That is why there is always a chance that an ODD child will remain angry and unexploited by History, stranded in a pool of social possibilities and evolutions. That is all the more why these people, the ODD people of unmaterialized potentials, the ODD people that their moment of glory will never arise during their lifetimes, the people that History forgot to capitalize upon, or already had a handful of better versions of them, enough Kevins and Hermanns to satisfy her needs of the time, the people who were omitted, the evolutionary-revolutionary leftovers, the people whose epoch was not ripe for them, or that were not ripe for their epoch, that is all the more why we should award their fruitless agonies with the full compensation of respect, under-standing and caring. It is the least we can do for people that are torn apart in emotional maelstroms only to be available when they are needed.

And I will not disagree that parents of ODD children may indeed lead intolerable lives. Then again, intolerable oddity in children often reflects intolerance in parents and societies. Societies that have turned over a great portion of freedoms and responsibilities to the experts' establishment, societies consisting of people who regard the humane aspects of life as burdening redundancies, people whose only commitments to life are work and consumption, silent acolytes of the mechanistic paradigm.

The progress of a civilization is not only defined by its technical or technological aspects and achievements, but predominantly by tolerance and understanding exhibited towards minorities; tolerance to difference is a safe guide regarding progress. In this "leave it to the expert" and "it's not my problem" culture, we have conquered the scientific audacity to create an artificial minority consistent of reactive children and we are arguing about the matter of course fact that children, a lot of them, are odd. And it is not about tolerance towards minorities anymore. Not until the right to be childlike is reinsti-tuted among children, not until the humane culture is reinsti-tuted, not until humanity is reinstituted. Define humane, Mr. ODD expert, define child, define normal and impose yourself serving definitions of a shallow science that was meant to explore the depths of the human soul to each and every one of us. No doubt, your private practice will gain clients, your profession will gain in stature, everyone will need your expert advice and you will create a society after your science's image. But you know, we still do possess an alternative, the ultimate one, the only one we really ever had. That is to live with people without definitions and learn and love and care and turn to the expert only when it is absolutely necessary and unavoidable. We have that much, Mr. Expert. It is our lives against your definitions. Is this a disorder also? Is being human a disorder? Because you seem to think that being a child is.

I have a dream. I have a dream that in this artificial world the ghost of humanitarianism will once again treat the globe with his beaten, burdened but still benign and thoughtful figure and present his difficult gifts to unwilling recipients. And once we unwrap this difficult package of a gift, we will discover life, the very essence of life beyond definitions, the direct life beyond confines. Wouldn't that be ODD???

But to get there we have first to follow Thomas Szasz's aphorism:

"Child psychology and child psychiatry cannot be reformed. They must be abolished."

# Chapter 6

# On the legality of drugs

*We are a drug pushing culture. And though we are pushing drugs to such an extent that we even treat drug addiction with replacement drugs like methadone, we culturally reject the use of drugs that have been culturally accepted and well tolerated for centuries. Loren Mosher described precisely this fundamental hypocrisy: "Unfortunately, APA reflects, and reinforces, in word and deed, our drug dependent society. Yet it helps wage war on "drugs". "Dual diagnosis" clients are a major problem for the field but not because of the "good" drugs we prescribe. "Bad" ones are those that are obtained mostly without a prescription."[162] This hypocrisy has deprived us of some substances that could give us some leverage over medical conditions we are failing to handle or even soothe. Though cocaine and its properties were praised and avidly consumed by 19th century psychiatrists, other, less harmful drugs were marginalized and discredited. Cannabis, for example, possesses unique painkilling properties and its therapeutic use could benefit thousands of patients living with acute or chronic pain, yet an inapprehensive social and moral stigma has been adhered to it, obstructing its therapeutic use. This culture is without a doubt a drug culture. The question is not whether it is pushing drugs but rather, whose drugs is it pushing.*

## a) Why doctors will give you only half-truths about...
### The Therapeutic Use of Cannabis

Cannabis has been with us for thousands of years and it has served us well. We depended on her to make clothes, ropes, to take some of the pain and stress away and sometimes even to float away from everyday's life worries into the unexplored space between words and ideas. Though recreational use of cannabis is not supported or suggested by the writer, the therapeutic use of cannabis is an altogether different issue.

The use of cannabis has been for the most of human history well accepted both culturally and medically.

Cannabis demonization was motivated by social prejudices and racial discrimination. In the early 20th century it was used to barricade the US from Mexican immigrants and later on from African American Jazz Musicians and the "evil" and "immoral" culture they were generating. Cannabis illegalization was promoted by Randolph Hearst who did not want cannabis as an antagonist in the paper business, and pharmaceutical companies who did not want to compete with a cheap and easily accessed – even homegrown painkiller.[163] As it is now, back then arguments did not have to be truthful to win over the support and sympathy of public opinion. They only had to appear credible and use fear and loathing to appeal not to the intellect but rather to the most primitive part of human nature. Even when people are unable to respond and conform to reason they can easily understand and comply to fear.

Today, thousands of otherwise law-abiding citizens are imprisoned as common criminals and thousands of patients are denied the therapeutic benefits of cannabis because of a social stigma that was adhered to it and a prohibitory culture which was, is and will be contradicting personal rights and freedom of choice.

Cannabis is not harmless. With the exception of side effects related not to cannabis itself but to respiratory problems associated with smoking, most of them are mild and fleeting. Still cannabis use may have some more severe implications like worsening the progression of liver fibrosis, triggering psychotic episodes,[164] causing subtle immune suppression.[165] But even some of these side effects can be turned into diagnostic and more easily therapeutic opportunities: cannabis-induced psychotic episodes have been suggested to have prognostic psychiatric value,[166] whereas the endocannabinoids' system immunomodulatory properties can inaugurate a whole new chapter in autoimmune disease therapeutics: the cannabinoid system in the central nervous system has been shown to regulate autoimmune inflammation, implying possible cannabinoid manipulation and treatment of multiple sclerosis![167] Cannabinoids are also being investigated for the treatment of other autoimmune disorders and allergies.[168] The active component of cannabis, $\Delta^9$-tetrahydrocannabinol (THC) has been found to inhibit the formation of "Alzheimer's plaques", slowing or possibly halting the progression of this virtually untreatable debilitating disease. According to the research team:

> Compared to currently approved drugs prescribed for the treatment of Alzheimer's disease, THC is a considerably superior inhibitor of $A\beta$ aggregation, and this study provides a previously unrecognized molecular mechanism through which cannabinoid molecules may directly impact the progression of this debilitating disease.[169]

Another study exhibited nerve growth promotion in the hippocampus of rats induced by the combination of high dosages of a synthetic cannabinoid alongside with the endocannabinoid anandamide.[170] Cannabis compounds have also shown a potential in the inhibition of lung (in vitro and animal models),[171] breast[172] and brain cancer. In brain cancer especially, THC promoted cancer cell autophagy leaving healthy cells intact.[173]

A brand new brave world of cannabinoid therapeutic possibilities and options lies ahead of us. Cannabis is also invaluable in chronic or drug-resistant pain management and general quality of living of patients with chronic health conditions. Despite the mild cannabis-induced immune suppression that is probably a counter-indication for AIDS patients, cannabis use was found to be beneficial both in AIDS anorexia and in AIDS related neuropathic pain.[174][175] Cannabis use has been shown to be beneficial also in nausea (especially drug-resistant cancer-chemotherapy induced nausea), vomiting, weight loss, premenstrual syndrome. Antioxidant properties have also been attributed to it.

After the illegalization of cannabis, medicalization happened to it. Instead of licensing patients in need of cannabis to even grow it at controlled amounts for personal therapeutic use, cannabis became a drug-industry property and cannabinoid compounds such as Nabinol, Marinol and Sativex that don't have the much-wanted immediate symptom relieving effects that the inhalation of vaporized cannabis possesses have been promoted as legal medical forms of cannabis. Who's next? Tea, chamomile, peppermint?

The benefit/risk ratio of cannabinoid compounds and of cannabis herself is very attractive and superior to that of other drugs employed to treat severe medical conditions. Cannabis appears to be "a miraculous" multitask therapeutic agent and its therapeutic use should be and would be heralded by scientists, patients and relatives worldwide. Instead, the social and legal stigma that has been attributed to her has inhibited relative research. It is once again a matter of politics against science, of prejudice against reason, of myths against facts. Who in his right mind would compare or downsize Alzheimer's disease or cancer or chronic drug-resistant pain, or multiple sclerosis to the side effects of cannabis use?

The hundreds of therapeutic applications, implications and possibilities of cannabis, even in conditions that there are no attractive, or not so effective or no therapeutic alternatives at all leaves us in awe of the extent to which human stupidity and stubbornness, political and financial mannerism and indecency, scientific cowardice and subjugation are halting medical progress.

*b) Why doctors will give you only half-truths about...*
## Antioxidants and Not Methadone Alone for the Rehabilitation of Addicts

Which expert can you believe, especially when they all appear so sincere? What will your doctor tell you, if you are an addict who wants rehabilitation?

Scientists are taught during their career to always be critical and analytical of the information presented to them and to always keep an open mind and to never get attached to the absolute truth of any theory. A safe bet is to regard the "truth" as the "best working hypothesis" of the day or the one that makes the logic practical and beneficial while seeking more information through research studies. The same applies to approaches to interventions for heroin addicts, rather than stick to a particular dogma as the absolute form of truth that must exclude all else, however compelling and logical.

Addiction is considered a medical illness with related psychological and social dimensions. Narcotics abuse creates problems for the body as it progress from experimental to addictive use for some people. This process occurs more quickly for some people than it does for others. During life, 98% of a dose of opiate is in the tissues; as the tissues of the body degenerate and break down, much of it will return to the bloodstream.[176] Such redistribution is less of a problem than for other drugs.[177]

Drug addiction is a pathological condition and can lead to the suppression of the immune system. Additionally, since drug metabolism generates free radicals in the body, the natural antioxidant levels can decline over time depending on the type of drug, the amount of drug abuse and on the individual's nutrition. Over time, oxidative damage begins to take its toll on general health and well-being and behavior. Drugs known to cause addiction include illegal drugs as well as prescription or over-the-counter drugs and the addictive potency of drugs varies from substance to substance, and from person to person.

The basic mechanisms by which different substances activate the reward system are as described above, but vary slightly among drug classes.[178]Whether they are depressants or stimulants, they disturb or disrupt the pathway involving dopamine produced in the brain that is part of the healthy reward system associated with behavior. Some drugs can cause disruption in the serotonin pathway as well, including its biosynthesis.

Depressants such as alcohol, barbiturates, and benzodiazepines work by increasing the affinity of the GABA receptor for its ligand – GABA. Narcotics such as morphine and heroin work by mimicking endorphins—chemicals produced naturally by the body which have effects similar to dopamine—or by disabling the neurons that normally inhibit the release of dopamine in the reward system. These substances typically facilitate relaxation and pain relief.

Stimulants such as amphetamines, nicotine, and cocaine increase dopamine signaling in the reward system either by directly stimulating its release or by blocking its absorption. These substances tend to cause heightened alertness and make one feel energetic. They produce a pleasant feeling called euphoria which is known as a high. Later this high wears off leaving the user feeling depressed. The depressing feeling sometimes makes the addict want more of the drug to get high again as a way to get out of depression but it can only worsen the situation and the addiction.

In both cases, healthy biochemistry that regulates behavior can be severely altered with ensuing pathological changes in long-term users of drugs and narcotics. In both cases, addicts want more of the drug or want it daily or regularly and dependency can develop into abuse.

Drug addiction as a disorder involves the progression of acute drug use to the development of drug-seeking behavior. It comes with the vulnerability to relapse and the decreased or slowed ability to respond to naturally rewarding stimuli. The Diagnostic and Statistical Manual of Mental Disorders, Fourth Edition (DSM-IV) has categorized three stages of addiction: preoccupation/anticipation, binge/intoxication, and withdrawal/negative effect. These stages are characterized, respectively, everywhere by constant cravings and preoccupation with obtaining the substance. With increasing tolerance in the initial phases there is more frequent use of more of the substance than necessary to experience the intoxicating effects followed by withdrawal symptoms and decreased motivation for life's normal activities.[179] The constant craving and preoccupation in obtaining the narcotic or substance is termed as drug-seeking behavior.

Drug-seeking behavior is a real problem rooted in biological changes in the addict. The mechanisms underlying drug addiction in the brain involves several areas of the brain and synaptic changes, or neuroplasticity, which occurs in these areas. Neuroplasticity is the putative mechanism behind learning and memory. It involves physical changes in the synapses between two communicating neurons, characterized by increased gene expression, altered cell signaling, and the formation of new synapses between the communicating neurons. When addictive drugs are present in the system, they appear to hijack this mechanism in the reward system so that motivation is geared towards procuring the drug rather than natural rewards.[180] Hence narcotics are commonly referred to as habit-forming drugs.

Drug addiction also raises the specter of another potential problem in the brain. First, neurogenesis decreases as a result of repeated exposure to addictive drugs but raises the issue of potential harmful effects on the development of new neurons in adults.

Detoxification is necessary to prepare patients for the treatment process. It is particularly important for those who have become dependent on alcohol and other CNS depressants, opiate drugs, and cocaine. Until the body is free of the effects of the drugs and the distorted thoughts and feelings they produce, it is difficult for recovery to begin.

Studies have shown that rapid relapse is likely to follow detoxification unless patients become engaged in additional treatment and transition services. Persons completing a detoxification program without continuing treatment are no more likely to succeed in reducing future drug use than persons achieving unassisted withdrawal.

The use of methadone has been well researched, and its effectiveness as part of the detoxification process for opiate drugs has been supported. However, many other drug treatments for alleviating withdrawal symptoms either have not been well researched or have resulted in contradictory findings. Thus, this is an area requiring additional medical research.

Your doctor may not tell you all about the use of methadone or other drugs which will be used on you as a replacement for the drug or drugs related to your addiction. Substitute drugs for other forms of drug dependence have historically been less successful than opioid substitute treatment but you have a right to know that the replacement drugs can cause the same addiction problem.

These forms of treatment include replacement drugs such as methadone or buprenorphine, used as a substitute for illicit opiate drugs.[181] Your doctor may not tell you that these are substitute therapies or that they are in fact an opiate replacement therapy – replacing one opiate for another. These are not real therapies because these drugs are themselves addictive.

Since opioid dependency can be extremely severe and these substitute therapies are about a way to stabilize opioid use and once stabilized, treatment enters maintenance or tapering phases. The tapering phases can be tricky because these substituted opiates such as methadone can cause the same neuroplastic changes in the brain. Hence, such therapies must be tightly regulated. Opiate replacement therapy is tightly regulated in methadone clinics by regulations or by a statutory act. In some countries, other opioid derivatives such as levomethadyl acetate, dihydrocodeine, dihydroetorphine and even heroin may be used as substitute drugs for illegal street opiates. Different drugs are used depending on the needs of the individual patient.[182]

Your doctor may not tell you what methadone is. Methadone, a synthetic narcotic analgesic compound, is the most commonly used form of pharmacotherapy for opiate drugs. Some literature states that it is medically safe and has few side effects. It produces a stable drug level and is not behaviorally or subjectively intoxicating. That is not true. It does, however, "block" or suppress the cravings for opiate drugs and does not produce euphoria, as heroin and other drugs do.

Methadone was originally developed by the Nazis during World War II. When the supply of opium was cut off, Nazi addicts like Hermann Goering (Commander in Chief of the Luftwaffe and Hitler's designated successor) wanted to avoid the possibility of withdrawal. He instructed the German drug companies to produce a wholly synthetic opiate that didn't need to rely on the poppy. The drug worked to alleviate withdrawal symptoms and its opiate effect also lasted a long time. As a result, methadone has become the drug of choice for doctors who are trying to help users manage their opiate dependency. Heroin wears off after a couple of hours, thus requiring several hits each day. Methadone, on the other hand, lasts anywhere between 24 and 72 hours, depending on the dose that you take and on your individual metabolism.

Among the various pharmacotherapies, methadone maintenance has been studied most thoroughly. Methadone maintenance is generally successful in meeting treatment goals. When appropriate doses of methadone are administered, heroin use decreases markedly. So, it is deemed an appropriate substitute for the more devastating heroin. However, "some (heroin) addicts readily admit that they prefer methadone as their drug of abuse."[183]

Methadone is now primarily used today for the treatment of narcotic addiction because the effects of methadone last longer than those of morphine-based drugs. Methadone's effects can last longer than 24 hours, thereby permitting administration only once a day in heroin detoxification and maintenance programs.

What advocates of methadone don't tell is this – methadone is a (synthetic opiate) narcotic that when administered once a day, orally, in adequate doses, can usually suppress a heroin addict's craving and withdrawal for 24 hours but patients can be as physically dependent on methadone as they were to heroin or other opiates, such as Oxycotin or Vicodin. Each time an addict uses heroin, there is a cycle consisting of intoxication, initially, followed by a period of normal mental functioning, which then yields to the discomfort of withdrawal and craving (flu-like symptoms with pain, anxiety and depression).

There are adverse reactions to methadone. Deaths occur more frequently at the beginning of treatment in methadone programs; they are usually a cause of excessive doses (i.e. erroneously estimated tolerance) and they are affected by concomitant diseases (hepatitis, pneumonia). Methadone generally entails the entire spectrum of opioid side effects, including the development of tolerance and physical and psychological dependence. Respiratory depressions are dangerous. The released histamines can cause hypotension or bronchospasms. Other symptoms are: constipation, nausea or vomiting, sedation, vertigo, edema.

The least common side effects of methadone are: anaphylactic reactions, hypotension causing weakness and fainting, disorientation, hallucinations, unstable gait, tremor, muscle twitching, myasthenia gravis. The risks include kidney failure and seizures.

Methadone and its metabolites can generate free radicals in the body and probably, and like heroin, may cause endothelial dysfunction and precipitate more health problems similar to those found in long-term smokers and associated with nitric oxide excess or lowering in the body.

As an opiate, regular use of methadone causes physical dependency – if you've been using it regularly (prescribed or not), once its use is stopped there will be an experience of withdrawal. The physical changes due to the drug are similar to other opiates (like heroin); suppressed cough reflex, contracted pupils, drowsiness and constipation. Some methadone users feel sick when they first use the drug. If you are a woman using methadone you may not have regular periods – but you are still able to conceive. Hence, advocates recommend a regulated dose.

Methadone is a long-acting opioid; it has an effect for up to 36 hours. Therefore a person who has switched to methadone will not withdraw for this period and it can remain in the body for several days. So, a daily (24 hour) intake of the methadone pill as a substitute for heroin covers the extended withdrawal time of 36 hours of methadone and the 8 hours for heroin. Hence, the regulated dose administration makes it appear that there is no withdrawal symptom in methadone use while it suppresses the craving for heroin. That is a bad approach, medically as well as on moral grounds. Your doctor will not tell you that the longer-acting methadone covers the withdrawal time for other opiates that have a shorter acting time. It is a masking mechanism and therefore it is known as a substitute therapy or replacement therapy, using a longer acting opiate to cover withdrawal time of shorter acting opiates – a very clever guise indeed. And drug replacement therapies also come disguised as "harm-reduction" therapy which has been positioned as the "best-working" hypothesis. Another way of looking at the "marketing" of drug-replacement therapies is that certain drugs are legalized for the addiction market by replacing the drugs or opiates that are made illegal.

Tolerance and addiction to methadone is a dangerous threat, as withdrawal results from the cessation of use. Many former heroin users have claimed that the horrors of heroin withdrawal were far less painful and difficult than withdrawal from methadone. Based on literature and analysis of mortality figures Dr. Russell Newcombe concluded that methadone programs as a form of harm-reduction possibly cause more victims than they prevent (Drs. Marcel Buster & Giel van Brussel, MD; Municipal Health Service Amsterdam).

One expert, Dr. George Fernandez, has said that governments must not take the warning lightly: if the use of methadone or other forms of drug substitution therapies (DST) were not adopted widely by the health authorities as soon as possible, the number of HIV/AIDS cases could shoot by 2015. People have been led to believe that a virus called the HIV causes AIDS and that the transmission of this virus must be stopped in the war against the HIV epidemic. A more perplexing issue in drug use, abuse and substitution is whether "HIV-AIDS spreads more slowly in methadone addicts and in persons using replacement drugs or replacement opiates."

What Dr. Gallo may have "isolated" is nothing more than broken proteins that have not been properly ingested by macrophages in stressed conditions as in the case of people with influenza, malaria etc and in people with a weakened immune system caused by free radical damage where the free radicals have been generated by immunotoxic drugs or narcotic abuse.

Heroin abuse generates free radicals in the body and its effects can be seen as early as in the third year of its abuse, primarily in the brain. Once it starts to initiate free radical chain reactions, the free radicals are produced in sufficient numbers to cause pain when it's hallucinatory and the pain blocking effect begins to wear off in about eight hours after taking the "shot". Heroin can cause feelings of depression, which may last for weeks. Attempts to stop using heroin can fail simply because the pain of the withdrawal can be overwhelming, causing the addict to use more heroin in an attempt to overcome these symptoms. That is the vicious trap of heroin that must be broken in order to help the heroin addict recover and progress to wellness.

Free radicals are unstable, destructive oxygen atoms. They are short of an electron in one of the orbits and are thus highly unstable. They will rob electrons from molecules nearby to gain stability. This process of robbing electrons initiated by radicals injure the body's healthy molecules by stealing electrons to replace their missing electrons to balance themselves and the process is called oxidative damage or oxidative injury. In the process, the free radicals injure cell membranes and leave damaged cells and tissues in their wake. This process is called oxidation and it's what makes iron rust and fruit turn brown.

The nausea, sweating, chills, convulsions, anxiety, nervousness, depression, headaches, hallucinations, diarrhea, restlessness/sleep disturbances, shaking (uncontrolled) are all caused by disruptions to normal and healthy biochemistry by excess free radicals and endothelial dysfunction while at a later stage, the chronic fatigue is due to mtDNA depletion caused by free radical damage to mitochondrial processes and muscular pains begins to appear as symptoms. This free radical avalanche may progress to further weakening of the immune system and opportunistic infections may take root and we have a picture of AIDS – all caused by the ravaging and extensive damage by free radicals over a few years.

Oxidative injury to cell walls renders them more vulnerable to penetration by pathogens, including viruses, and heroin addicts are therefore at a higher risk to opportunistic infections while the increasing free radical population in their bodies decreases their tolerance to opiates. The rapid depletion of antioxidants by the increasing loads of free radicals generated by heroin and its metabolites results in rapid loss of tolerance to heroin.

Research investigating vitamin C's ability to aid in detoxification following alcohol and drug abuse is one of the most promising avenues of research being pursued today. In a highly promising and well-known mechanism, vitamin C is able to prevent the oxidative damage caused by alcohol metabolism in the following manner: vitamin C donates electron to the SOD-catalase-glutathione antioxidant system that, in a step-wise fashion, converts the excess-oxygen free radicals generated during drug/alcohol metabolism into water and oxygen, making the SOD-catalase-glutathione detox reactions more effective in preventing oxidative damage. The body has an ascorbate-dependent detoxification system which is more active than the alcohol dehydrogenase or Cytochrome P450 microsomal systems. In one study, whereas half the alcohol-dosed guinea pigs developed liver necrosis, none of the vitamin C-treated animals developed liver damage. Increasing glutathione in the biological system through dietary intake and supplements provides additional help. Fruit and vegetable juices are therefore essential as part of the rehabilitative therapy, including their extracts in nano-form for rapid detox.

In humans, vitamin C was demonstrated to significantly enhance alcohol clearance, and even to effect substantial improvements in behavior, especially motor coordination. And, since Vitamin C reduces fat accumulation in the liver following alcohol consumption, it appears that Vitamin C may protect against direct damage to the liver from alcohol. There are several new studies that show that vitamin C intake before alcohol consumption reduces the risk to the brain and the liver which is primarily on account of its role as an antioxidant, while the breakdown of alcohol in the liver produces metabolites that have free radical generating capacity.

Smokers have below-normal levels of vitamin C – as much as 40% lower in pack-a-day smokers. Cigarettes smoke contains excessive amounts of free radicals that effectively deplete vitamin C in the body. After it has lost or donated its electron to the free radicals in the smoke it is broken down and excreting it much faster than normal. Studies show that people exposed to second-hand smoke also need extra vitamin C.

There is also strong indication that vitamin C relieves withdrawal symptoms in heroin addicts, something that should be naturally expected, bearing in mind that it is a free radical scavenger; but it is submitted that the treatment of withdrawal symptoms will be more effective by using a combination of natural antioxidants and to help put the heroin or methadone addict on the road to wellness. Alpha-lipoic acid and ligands from vegetables is an effective biochelator that can bind drug residues and help to remove them from the biological system through excretion. The drug residues must be effectively and safely removed from the synapses and the process that leads to neuroplastic changes. Drugs and opiates that are used as replacements to the drugs and opiates that have caused the addiction cannot do that and can have cumulative effects as well. The answer lies in using biomolecules of a different nature that support healthy biochemistry.

Wellness is defined as the constant and deliberate effort to stay healthy and achieve the highest potential for well-being. It is a life-long process of becoming aware of and identifying areas that need improvement in one's life, and making choices to attain goals of a higher level of health and well-being. Physical wellness is thought of as the ability to carry out daily tasks, to develop cardio-respiratory and muscular fitness, maintain proper nutrition & healthy body fat levels. Avoid abusing alcohol or drugs and tobacco products.

Studies have shown nicotine to be as addictive as heroin and cocaine. Tar is the dark substance that actually carries the nicotine to the lungs. Along with the nicotine it also carries the long list of other chemicals: Benzene and Radon. Benzene is highly toxic because it generates large amounts of free radicals in the body. Today benzene is also an additive to petrol.

It is quite obvious that the taking of methadone as a substitute for heroin or other opiate addiction will require tapering and this phase must be properly supported by a high dietary intake of fruit-vegetable juices, but the administration of rapidly acting antioxidants made from natural and edible sources, which are generally regarded as safe, are a preferred option, more so if it can be also shown that it can also build up the immune system, prevent opportunistic infections and reduce the craving for opiates, cigarettes and alcohol.

Any government must quickly discard its old methods, including the "methadone-harm-reduction" approach and consider a logical paradigm shift to support a new study that would use a rapidly acting antioxidant spray and a diet rich in natural antioxidants to eliminate the pain of withdrawal symptoms, reducing the craving for opiates from day to day and put the addict on the path to wellness for harm-reduction, as a goal through replacement therapies is not good enough. They must be augmented with a high dietary intake of antioxidants and other antioxidant therapies must be used.

Drug addiction is a complex brain condition characterized by compulsive drug craving, seeking, and use that persist even in the face of severe adverse consequences. For most people, drug addiction becomes chronic, with relapses possible even after long periods of abstinence. As a chronic, recurring illness, addiction may require continued treatments to increase the intervals between relapses and diminish their intensity. Treatment of such a complex problem cannot be achieved by drugs or drug substitution alone; and any integrated treatment must be tailored to individual needs to enable people with drug addiction to have a better chance to recover and lead productive lives.

# Chapter 7

# Towards a new public health model

*Since the times of Homo Farber, we have learned to replace or discard things that are not working anymore. For one reason or another we are not applying this wise practice to the current dysfunctional public health model. Why is that?*

## a) Why doctors will give you only half-truths about...
## The Death of Medicine

Demand for health care has put national health services under increasingly severe strain as the rise in cost of medicine is escalating. The situation is worst in countries without national health that depend on health insurance. In the United States, employer-sponsored health insurance premiums more than doubled between 1996 and 2006, 4 times the increase in wage;[184] and more and more people find themselves uninsured.

The US spent $2.2 trillion on health care in 2007; averaging $7421 per person, 16.2% of GDP, and nearly twice the average of other developed nations. Yet this most advanced and costly medical system in the world is the leading cause of death and injury to its citizens. Each year, some 2.2 million suffer from adverse drug reaction, 7.5 million undergo unnecessary medical and surgical procedures, and 8.9 million are unnecessarily hospitalized. In 2001, the medical system killed 783,936, when 699,697 died from heart disease and 553,251 from cancer.[185]

The health care system is failing the world over.[186] [187] Health journalist and author Nick Regush summed it up starkly:

Medicine, as we know it, is dying...The disease is caused by conflict of interest, tainted research, greed for big bucks, pretentious doctors and scientists, lying, cheating, invasion by the morally bankrupt marketing automatons of the drug industry, derelict politicians and federal and state regulators... As a journalist, it has become very plain to see how little anything the medical Establishment does these days can be trusted or taken at face value. Press conferences, journal articles, symposia – all are geared to spike and obfuscate the truth, to hide red flags from the public and to bulk up the shares of investors in the companies that are promoting the science and the researchers. [188]

## Domo did it

Regush and others have correctly identified the proximate causes conspiring in the death of medicine. But those are all symptomatic of a deeper cause, the obsolete model that dominates not just medicine, but the whole of our lives. Let's call it Domo for short.

Domo runs our economy, our industries; it lurks behind our political, social, and educational institutions, its tendrils woven into the fabric of our lives. We accept it unthinkingly, mistaking it for the ineluctable ultimate reality. Whenever something goes wrong, we look for someone, something else to blame; leaving Domo looming larger and stronger than ever before.

Public debates on the causes and cures for AIDS,[189] GM foods,[190] mobile phones,[191] pesticides,[192] and more, are all in the service of Domo, because we leave it untouched in the process of destroying ourselves.

Isn't it time we blow the cover on Domo?

## Science of death vs. science of life, mechanism vs. organism

Domo is a seductively powerful view of the world as machine that can be taken apart, analyzed, controlled, and re-tooled to serve our every want, wish, and whim. It had ushered in the industrial revolution and shaped the subsequent history of our planet right up to the present multiple crises in the throes of climate change.

Scientific enquiry has its own momentum, however, and the mechanistic science of Domo was already becoming obsolete at the turn of the past century when the science of the organism emerged. I have outlined how Domo's economy of infinite unsustainable growth that depends on competition and profligate dissipation should be replaced with nature's own closed loop economy that minimizes wastes and thrives on reciprocity and co-operation.[193] This organic circular model applies especially to sustainable agroecological systems that can mitigate climate change while providing food and fuel security for all.[194]

Here, I shall sketch out how the science of the organism can replace Domo biology and revolutionize our understanding of health, and health care.

Domo's influence in biology has been the most profound and persistent. It presents the organism as a junkyard of molecular nuts and bolts subject to mechanistic principles of lock and key, push and pull, random collision, linear causation, controller versus controlled etc. Diseases are largely viewed as 'defects' in specific molecular mechanisms, and defined as such. This is the kind of thinking behind the human genome project that has all the signs of having run aground after decades of sequencing and dissecting genomes, and trying to identify the genetic defects that predispose individuals to different diseases.[195] Together with the physical laws of equilibrium thermodynamics and statistical mechanics, Domo biology is essentially a science of death that has virtually nothing to say about life.

Erwin Schrödinger's book, *What is Life?*[196] was one of the first critiques of the mechanistic representation of life. It is widely acclaimed for having predicted the genetic material DNA. Much less known and more significantly, it also predicted the molecular coherence of organisms discovered in my laboratory in 1992; which, too, has been largely ignored.

Living organisms have such a high degree of molecular coherence that they appear as dynamic liquid crystal displays under the polarizing microscope geologists use for identifying crystals. If you have a chance to marvel at these images, you can have a unique insight of what it is to be alive.[197]

The science of the organism is predicated on a radical wholeness or coherence of the living system, which profoundly transforms our view of health and disease.

*Quantum coherent liquid crystalline organism works by intercommunication*

The wholeness of the organism transcends the age-old opposition between "top-down" and "bottom-up" explanations, or holist *versus* the reductionist approach in Domo biology. Instead, every single level is working together simultaneously, right down to individual molecules whose motions are so correlated in the tissues and cells that they make living organisms look like liquid crystal displays. Watch the videos of live organisms set to music in the Quantum Jazz DVD,[198] and notice how the most active organisms and the most active parts of organisms give the brightest most brilliant colors because they are also the most coherent.

In the healthy coherent organism, each single molecule is *intercommunicating* with every other; and each is as much in control as it is sensitive and responsive. There is no need for push and pull, because coherent energy is stored throughout the system, ready to be mobilized. This coherence explains why organisms *are* sensitive to the weak electromagnetic fields of the mobile phone and wireless networks saturating our environment,[199] especially because the organism uses electromagnetic fields and electric currents for intercommunication.

A convenient description for the wholeness of the organism is 'quantum coherence' extending over all modes of living activities, from very slow circadian or circa-annual rhythms to the ultrafast femto-second energy transfers between molecules; from the extremely local to the global. This hive of exquisitely coordinated activities is a 'quantum jazz'[200] performed over a musical range of 70 octaves, in which every player is improvising spontaneously and freely, yet keeping in tune and in step with the whole.

The most accessible evidence of the body-wide coherence of biological rhythms comes from the fractal and multifractal variations of the healthy heartbeat, which reflect an intricate phase correlation among all rhythms as the heart's own beat intermeshes and syncopates in symphony with the rest.[201] In contrast, the diseased heart that's no longer communicating with the body falls back on its intrinsic rhythm and becomes much more regular. This has opened up a whole new field of dynamic disease that can be diagnosed by mathematics, and possibly treated non-invasively by biofeedback techniques.[202] The coherent organism is a unity of brain and body, heart and mind, an undivided bundle of intellect and passion, flesh, blood, and sinew that lives life to the full, freely and spontaneously, attuned not just to the immediate environment, but the universe at large. This ideal coherent whole is also the ideal of health.

*Water is means, medium, and message*
Quantum jazz is possible because organisms *are* liquid crystalline; the 70% by weight of water making up the tissues and cells are an integral, necessary part of the liquid crystalline matrix that enables rapid intercommunication to take place, whereby the organism can function as a coordinated whole.

New research described in the latest edition of my book[203] show how this special biological water in tissues and cells provide the means, medium and message for intercommunication.

The liquid crystalline water is the ultimate source of protons

(H⁺) and electrons (e⁻), positive and negative charges that zap through cellular compartments, between cells and tissues and the most distant parts of the body, energizing the organism, instantaneously coordinating its metabolism, growth, and other vital functions.

The liquid crystalline water matrix pervades the entire organism from the extracellular connective tissues to the interior of every single cell. Special membrane proteins have water-filled channels that cross the cell membrane, acting as "proton wires" to transport protons in and out of the cell.[204] This same matrix transmits the heart's large pulsating electromagnetic field throughout the body, including the brain, which paces and intercommunicates with the myriad local rhythms.[205] Within the cell, it transmits the much higher frequency electromagnetic waves emitted by molecules that depend on specific frequencies to recognize one another and coordinate their actions even at a distance.[206] The liquid crystalline matrix converts pressure and heat into electricity (and *vice versa*), thereby coordinating the perfect movements of both voluntary and involuntary muscles that enable some people to be concert pianists, Olympic athletes, or kung fu masters. The thermoelectric and piezoelectric effects, typical of liquid crystals, may underlie the therapeutic effects of massage and other "subtle energy medicine"[207] possibly by restoring coherence to the body, as well as a balance of positive and negative charges.

Special water channels in confined spaces aligned by collagen fibers have the potential to serve as superconducting proton cables, being really many proton wires wound together,[208] and may well correspond to the acupuncture meridians of traditional Chinese medicine, as David Knight and I suggested in 1998.[209] The anatomical correlates of acupuncture meridians remain unknown to this day.[210] Intriguingly, water next to charged hydrophilic surfaces, which are everywhere within the organism, not only forms ordered liquid crystalline layers, but can also be charged up by light, infrared light at 3-100-nm being the most effective in expanding the ordered layers that become charged up like a battery.[211] This finding reinforces the emerging picture that water is the lead player in bioenergetics.[212] As Nobel Laureate Albert Szent-Gyorgyi remarked, water is "the mother of all life."[213]

*Gene medicine based on Domo genetics*
'Biologicals', genetically engineered protein drugs, the first of which was insulin, are now found to cause adverse events and death more frequently than synthetic chemical drugs.[214] This comes as no surprise, as genetic engineering is the epitome of Domo genetics that does not recognize the organic coherent whole where all genes and gene products are engaged in quantum jazz. You cannot just throw in an extra gene and hope it will slot into place like a missing logo piece.

Domo genetics was already superseded by the genetics of the fluid genome as the first biological was commercialized,[215] the fluid genome being part and parcel of the coherent organism perfectly attuned to its environment, constantly intercommunicating with it, altering gene expression and the genes themselves.

Decades of sequencing and dissecting the human genome in the hope of identifying genes for diseases have only served to confirm that the real causes of ill health are environmental and social.[216]

It is not the genetic messages encoded in genomic DNA, but environmentally-induced epigenetic modifications that overwhelmingly determine people's health and well-being. Early nutrition and parental care play a large role in an individual's physical and mental health,[217] and due attention must be paid to those aspects in delivering primary health care.

*Domo medicine must go, but basic research is needed for the new organic medicine*

Domo medicine is obsolete and doing more harm than good. That's why people are turning to complementary therapies, not all based on well-founded knowledge, however.

In May 2009, 67% in Switzerland voted in favor of a constitutional article for complementary medicine.[218] The Swiss vote reflects the growing importance of complementary medicine in Europe. Some 65% of Europeans report they have used complementary and alternative medicine, with 30–50% using it as self-support and 19 to 20% having seen a complementary or alternative medical practitioner in the past year.

In contrast to the growth in popularity of complementary medicine, the science of the organism that could underpin it has languished, being valiantly pursued by only a few pioneers such as Jim Oschman,[219] formerly a cell biologist.

I have outlined the basic physics of the organism and its potential connections to dynamic diseases and complementary therapies. A new "organic medicine" could combine the best in non-invasive, non-destructive approaches from both traditional medical systems and contemporary science that would also revitalize indigenous medicines in all cultures and provide affordable health care for all. This project is all the more urgent in view of the increase in disease burden forecast for times of climate change.

### b) Why doctors will give you only half-truths about...
### The Future of Medicine

Scientists are trained during their career to always be critical and analytical of the information presented to them and to always keep an open mind and to never get attached to the absolute truth of any theory. A safe bet is to regard the "truth" as the "best working hypothesis" of the day or the one that makes the data or findings logical, practical and beneficial while seeking more information through research. Quite often though, many people's mental development end by acquiring a professional degree and the skills to carry out procedures and methods or a practice and the mind, having anchored in a particular mindset, tends to operates within its confines.

One of the mindsets that is being radically altered through research in cellular biochemistry is the traditional pharmaceutical notion of one disease–one drug.

Long ago, it was discovered that sailors on long sea voyages suffered from a condition called scurvy that could be cured by consuming onions or oranges simply because it was caused by a drop in cellular function due to a chronic depletion of vitamin C. Natural vitamin C as an antioxidant promotes aerobic respiration in cells as it readily scavenges free radicals that cause oxidative stress on the Krebs cycle. Its severe depletion (below 60%) in the cell, over time, adversely affects optimal cellular function in all organs.

That original health science concept of natural vitamin C as a cure has been abandoned and replaced with the idea of giving patients a "pharmaceutically-prescribed" drug, even if that means a synthetic antioxidant. And several new synthetic antioxidants have received patents and will become part of "pharmaceutically prescribed" practice in modern medicine in the years ahead. One of the characteristics of allopathic medicine is that it is patent-driven.

Excess free radicals, whether of endogenous origin produced by metabolic reactions in the cell or from exogenous sources such as from cigarette smoke from exhaust fumes or toxic drugs or during the breakdown of chemicals such as alcohol in the liver, can exert oxidative stress on the Krebs cycle and/or mitochondrial activity in cells, especially in persons who have a low intake of antioxidants and bioavailable minerals in their diet. That oxidative stress can interfere with cellular biochemical reactions and lower cellular function and over time or under severe oxidative stress cellular function may become impaired, leading to disease conditions.

Free radicals are ions that have an unpaired electron and are therefore positively charged. They are highly unstable and "rob" electrons from other biomolecules in the body and that initiates free radical chain reactions. Proteins and other molecules that have been damaged by free radicals can cause degenerative disease states in the body.

One of the most reactive species of free radicals is the hydroxyl ion which reacts in one nanosecond and excess hydroxyl ions produce hydrogen peroxide that inactivates the enzymes involved in the Krebs cycle, lowering cellular energy output and may eventually shut it down leading to death of the cell or abnormal functioning of the cell.

In biochemical terms, health can be defined as the optimal functioning of cells. When a significant number of cells begin to function at levels below the optimal levels, cellular energy output decreases and one feels lethargic or fatigue sets in. If the antioxidant and micronutrient levels in those cells remain low, then disease conditions begin to manifest. In such situations aging may also proceed at an accelerated rate.

Prolonged oxidative stress depletes antioxidants in the cells and tissues creating an unhealthy state in the cellular environment that eventually leads to oxidative injury. Oxidative injury is said to have occurred when certain and clear symptoms appear such as lower production of antibodies by the immune system due to oxidative suppression of the immune system by excess free radicals. Naturally, if through some intervention, impaired or diminished cellular function can be restored to its optimal level, health is restored.

Some examples of oxidative injury include oxidative injury to the cell membranes leading to retention of sodium ions in the cells or migration of magnesium ions out of the cells and into the bloodstream.

Another example of oxidative stress is oxidative stress in smokers on cells in the arterial endothelium causing them to produce excess nitric oxide that in turn acts as free radical stressor associated in a cluster of diseases such as diabetes, ED, MS, cardiovascular disease. In all of these cases, there is depletion of the body's natural antioxidants including coenzyme Q10, glutathione and other selenoproteins and alpha-lipoic acid. If excess nitric oxide is induced in a pregnant woman, whether by smoke or drugs, it passes through the placenta and it could interfere with metabolic processes in the fetus and could cause developmental defects in the fetus, such as "hole-in-heart" etc.

Research has also shown that cells under oxidative stress, as in smokers, become impaired in their cellular function as indicated by lower production of hormones and other protein molecules. In a disease condition, as such in cancers, a particular protein may not be manufactured in the cell due to severe depletion of the natural antioxidants in those cells.

Research has proven that when the natural antioxidant enzyme levels in cells drop below 80% the cell dies and when the natural vitamin C level in white blood cells drops below 60% it cannot function properly in its cytotoxic role that kills pathogens. During phagocytosis, the white blood cell resorts to anaerobic respiration to produce a sudden burst of free radicals directed at the pathogen and the hydrogen peroxide formed, inactivates the enzymes in the bacterial cell but it requires excess natural vitamin C to stop the anaerobic respiration initiated to produce free radicals that are cytotoxic to the bacterial cell.

A good example of a condition caused by very rapidly acting free radicals is when a bee sting causes immediate pain and there is very rapid swelling around the sting. Bee venom contains free radicals and it generates free radicals very rapidly. Most allopathic drugs and heavy metal ions do not produce such rapid reactions.

The common factor in antibiotics and almost all of allopathic drugs, anti-parasitic drugs, chemotherapy drugs and radiation is that they all generate free radicals in the body, in particular the hydroxyl ion which is cytotoxic to both the pathogen or cancer cells as well normal cells, and when in excess causes the so-called complications from drug use. Practically every drug has its benefit-risk profile. In contrast, cellular medicine aims to first remove the oxidative stress (through the use of antioxidants) on cells followed by providing micronutrients in bioavailable form so that the improving cellular function will enable aerobic energy output as well as increase the natural antioxidant enzyme levels, which further improve cellular function.

Many allopathic drugs are blockers or inhibitors and while they may be effective in blocking a pathway that appears connected to a disease state, such as high (bad cholesterol) LDL, it may also block the pathway that produces an antioxidant enzyme such as coenzyme Q10. Statin drugs used in cardiovascular disease end up in reducing the coenzyme Q10 levels in heart muscle, thereby increasing the risk to the heart. Coenzyme Q10 is essential in the pathway that yields cellular energy to muscle cells and it is also an antioxidant. Nature, very wisely, carved a double role for such biomolecules, which means that they participate in cell biochemistry, physiological roles and protect the cells in the advent of oxidative stress, and cellular medicine would naturally aim to devise interventions that would increase the overall Q10 levels in people with cardiovascular disease.

These case scenarios highlight the inherent conflict of allopathic medical practice with cellular biochemistry. Some systems of medicine aim to boost the immune function or the blood antioxidant levels etc, whereas in contrast the allopathic system of drug use allows the use of drugs that are immunosuppressive or immunotoxic.

Most allopathic drugs especially the chemo-drugs and AZT are highly toxic. Its earlier label classified it as a poison and toxic if inhaled. Ironically, today it is prescribed after a person is "tested" positive for antibodies. Such drugs can generate large amounts of the hydroxyl ion in the body and cause oxidative stress on cellular function and produce complications in organs, and in excess or prolonged use, causes cells to die. The chemo-drugs do not discriminate between normal cells and cancer cells. There must be a legal requirement for doctors to explain and make patients understand the devastating effects of chemo-drugs, which should not be referred to as medications or medicines. At the very least, there must be a legal requirement for the doctor to explain the benefit-risk situation to all cancer patients before the commencement of treatment by chemo-drugs or treatment by radiation.

Treatment by such toxic drugs depletes the natural antioxidants in the body and weaken or suppress or otherwise destroy the body's immune system or impair or diminish cellular function and hence there must be a requirement to test for the serum levels of antioxidants before the commencement of the treatments with toxic drugs and these levels must be regularly monitored during the treatment period.

The fundamental need for such tests is that serum levels or cellular levels of the natural antioxidant enzymes are predictive of cell death and death of the patient. Finally, when a patient, who was treated with toxic drugs, dies during the treatment these tests must be carried out to determine if the death was caused by the cancer disease or the oxidative stress caused by the treatment. In a developed society, people have a right to such critical information.

Some societies use herbs that have biomolecules that rapidly generate the hydroxyl ion that kills parasites and research is being carried out to asses their therapeutic use in malaria etc, but these herbs are also rich in natural antioxidants including vitamins and bioavailable minerals.

Clearly, allopathic medicine is a system of its own; there is no case for integrating the allopathic system with the cellular medicine and allopathic doctors should be allowed to continue with their system. It is the only system taught in medical schools and they currently form the establishment.

There is, however, an opportunity for initiating a paradigm shift. It is for the people to fight for the use of their tax funds to establish medical schools that train medical students in all the advancements in diagnostic science and imaging, medical procedures, ER medicine, free radical biochemistry and disease, clinical nutrition and the role of antioxidants in restoring biochemical pathways in cellular function in order to restore optimal cellular function and health. In a developed society people must be given a choice to opt for treatments that affect their health and quality of life.

Scientists have made many contributions that are being applied in the allopathic system, and within the allopathic system medical professionals have made great strides in life-saving procedures and practices including life-support systems. Researchers in many fields have contributed to medical science that may have benefited people like you and me. I applaud all the life-saving roles that allopathic medicine has made thus far and all that progress and benefit to humanity can be culled for application in other systems especially in cellular medicine.

The real case is, therefore, not one of integrating other treatment concepts with the allopathic practice, but quite obviously taking only those advances in medical science that augment the practice of any alternative medicine such as a system for the application of antioxidants to restore biochemical pathways in cells in order to promote optimal functioning of the target cells or tissues or organs of system.

Allopathic medical practice has evolved around the use of drugs. It cannot be integrated into any of the other systems.

Medical specialists can then continue prescribing medications containing benzene derivatives, petrochemicals, paraffins, propylene glycol, parabens etc, and sprays that contain alcohol, isopropyl derivatives and propellants such as isobutane, propane and butane and synthetic antioxidants. Allopathic medical practice should be allowed unhindered with their use of free radical generating drugs and inhibitors and radiation but it must not come to pass, that in the year 2020, health is still the monopoly of allopathic doctors.

Development is about making informed decisions and educated choices. I hope that advances in biotechnology will parallel changes in the type of developments that enable the making of informed choices and to support such progress in our society; education in health science is but an imperative.

## c) Why doctors will give you only half-truths about...
## Re-humanizing Medicine

In the old world there were three types of "health practitioners" that historically might have been discrete or intertwined. The doctor as we have come to know him, dealing with the physical body, removing poisons and toxins; the "witch doctor", dealing with the "astral body", removing bad influences of the spirit world; and the healer dealing with the "soul", reuniting all elements of self in harmony.

Modern medicine, being an industry that creates doctors who are highly-trained specialists, technicians of the body, has shifted away from the ancient perceptions of healing and treatment, crystallizing and adopting only the mechanical aspect of it.

It is true that we don't need witch doctors anymore. We have alternative rock to get rid of the "bad spirits", no need for such a type of an atavistic medicine.

But the healer is a class of "doctor" that we are in desperate need of. We tore the universe into pieces in order to understand it a bit better but we never bothered to glue it or stitch it back together.

We did the same thing with the human entity. Tore it to

pieces, understood the function of organs, the role of cell populations but, hey we forgot something along the way: the sick person standing across is a glorious undivided person, not just a sum of organs arranged by anatomy.

Mind, body and emotion interactions play a tremendous role in the healing process. Stress, self-rejection or rejection from others, violence physical or emotional, hatred and even love can deeply injure a person and affect its body-soul state of being. In fact, if we were to evaluate each and every factor, biological, environmental, emotional, genetical, each and every aspect and parameter of the microcosm and the macrocosm, then, even with the most powerful computer, we would be unable to determine a single characteristic, to get one simple answer, to make one simple diagnosis. We do not possess the science of the Cosmos yet, we don't have the ultimate calculating instrument nor do we possess the ultimate machine of data gathering. Laplace's demon died long ago. But determinism didn't, at least not in the medical science. It guides us; it is through it that medical decisions are taken. And needless to say, it does not suffice.

So what are we left with? Some medical knowledge, in fact lots of it, granted. It is not enough though. Though we discarded them as useless, we are still equipped with two crucial human quantities: passion and compassion, motivation stemming from the very depths of self and of "the others".

I can hardly think of any great scientific figure the last four centuries that wasn't driven by a burning passion to discover "the truth" of the cosmos or by a childhood curiosity to discover how the cosmos actually works.

I can hardly think of any great medical figure throughout history that wasn't driven by passion to serve his fellow man, to ease the pain and the hardships of life. I can hardly think of any great medical figure that wasn't driven by the Love of man and life. I can hardly think of any great doctor, from Hippocrates to Semmelweis that wasn't driven by compassion, by a feeling of belonging and offering.

Modern science has been systematically sterilized from passion, presenting it as a scientific limpness, as a liability. In its stead, it promoted the idea of a science highly distilled, purified from the besetting sins of human character and the grandiose bloomers and feats of the human spirit. We decided to disassociate science from scientists, to dehumanize science and put it into auto-pilot, to industrialize it and to create hordes of lab rats, of specialists who are no more than the scientific instruments they use and the funds they receive. Yes, the science we produce and encourage, follow and serve is the science of lab rats, not the science of men. Here you go, take another cup of espresso science.

Granted, passion often leads to mistakes. But there no is true learning without mistakes. We, the sentient creatures, learn from our mistakes and it is the safest way for us to learn.

There is no science without sentience. If there were, microscopes and telescopes and computers would produce science. But they can't. Science is of the humans and it should at least be humane.

And passion does not necessarily contradict objectivity.

Psychiatry typically "robbed" her followers and practitioners from one of the greatest qualities of the human being: Empathy. The process has to be free of transference, in the same fashion that the confessor has to appear immune to sin or temptation. Both disciplines presented morally strong, male yet asexual archetypes unaffected by human passion and thus not affectionate. That is pretty much also the archetype of modern science: morally strong, male yet asexual, impassionate, flawless, unaffected and not affectionate, free from the primordial sin of being human and feeling the feelings of self and other. Yes, science is a Swiss watch. If that is so, why is it missing the historic momentum over and over again?

This patriarchic hypocrisy of the infallible science has

217

produced horrors invisible to the naked, untrained eye.

We thought we purified science. We didn't, we couldn't. What we did was to refuse science of its humanity. That way we forced all human vices to mimic scientific discipline and method and dig their way into scientific leadership. By thinking of science as impregnable, intact by definition and infallible we succumbed to mortal sins far more dangerous than passion: arrogance and indifference, the sense that things could and would work just fine without us tending for them. Science from an adventurous and open process became a politically and financially controlled calculating machine, a self-fulfilled prophesy: feed it the data you want and it will give the results you crave for. Once science used to exemplify and theorize using controlled conditions experiments. Now itself has become a typical example of a full-scale financially controlled experiment. Parasites that were trained to become part of the scientific mechanism, or simply understood how it worked or saw the parallelisms with other systems, took over it and took advantage of it to serve their own agendas.

Soon, the garden of science became infested with weeds and parasites and turned unproductive, a self-serving mechanism where its sole interest was to perpetuate itself even at the expense of others. In times that science is too weak; it is employed into stronger parasitic mechanisms that exploit not its actual productivity but rather the potential it still holds to produce ideas, innovation and social usefulness.

Science suffered from the same sickness that brought global economy to its knees from 2008 to 2010: it stopped serving any purposes other than self-interest, it was stripped of real values that were replaced by virtual ones and it disassociated profit from social usefulness.

You see it happening so often in nature, one could say it is a natural law: once an organism looses self-efficiency or looses the ability to produce, it becomes parasitic or predatory and turns to other organisms to feed, to sustain itself.

Science used to be essential to society and to civilization as plants are to ecosystems and life. And in a sense, science is a photosynthetic organism. It turns energy (thoughts and ideas) into matter (technology) and food (applications, products and services). That was before it was taken over by cliques of "scientific" organizations and priesthoods and by the mobs of finance.

The more predators there are the more the remaining productive organisms are targeted. In such an environment, the productive species of science and economy are left with few options, few survival strategies:

a) Turn parasitic or predatory themselves.
b) Develop a parasitic-like or predatory-like or environment-like mimicry thatconfuses their hunters. Once safe, the mime can go on with his normal productive life circle: the "chameleon" survival strategy.
c) Develop unpleasantness or appear inedible: the skunk survival strategy.
d) Become poisonous or thorny: the poison ivy and porcupine survival strategies.
e) Play dumb: the ostrich survival strategy.
f) Play dead: the opossum survival strategy.

It is obvious that no matter what strategy is followed by the remaining productive species, the more predatory a system becomes the more effort, time and energy is devoted to survival and maintenance and the less productive the system tends to be.

Following destructive, cost ineffective and energy consuming policies, we are now facing the need to turn to the bountiful alternative sources of energy. But we haven't yet been forced to address the same class of problems regarding science, and especially medicine, a mechanism that is mutating into a destructive, cost ineffective and energy consuming organism.

From the self-interested, earth-centric science of today we

must be at least as brave as Copernicus and turn more helio-
centric, that is, turn to light and clarity for energy and
sustainment in industry and science. Without the light of the sun
and the light of the intellect, we, the surface dwellers that
achieved greatness by looking upwards, to the sky, to stars and
beyond, will turn into eternal coal and oil digging rats, or Nobel
and fund-seeking lab rats.

Medicine must be restored as the science of man for man and
stop feeding on diseased or dead flesh.

"If only there was a pandemic, that would be great for
business" said the cynical proprietor of the funeral parlor, to the
his Big Pharma CEO high school buddy.

"What a great idea! What didn't I think of it before!" the CEO
exclaimed in amazement.

This imaginary dialog might sound like a joke but the fact that
death and modern medicine go hand in hand is not funny at all.

### d) Why doctors will give you only half-truths about...
**The Final Public Health Solution**

Some decades ago, Ivan Illich, an important intellectual,
referred to iatrogenesis, that is, to adverse effects and complications resulting not from health problems but from medical intervention itself. I guess back in the 1970s lots of people involved in
Big Pharma must have thought: "What a great idea! Why didn't
we think of it earlier?"

Since then, disease mongering has become an ever more
popular marketing strategy for companies and health professionals. Find a disease and you come up with a new market.
Devise one and you still come up with a new market. Call it an
epidemic and you expand your market even further. That as was
sound advice as any, and Big Pharma with a little help from its
lackeys were quick to catch up with that innovative notion of
artificial diseases opening new marketing horizons.

But today the situation has gotten completely out of hand.

And it is not only because of the pressure exerted by Big Pharma to science and society. The entire health care system is falling apart.

According to a 2003 report by the Nutrition Institute of America:

> New information has been presented showing the degree to which Americans have been subjected to injury and death by medical errors. The results of seven years of research reviewing thousands of studies conducted by the NIA now show that medical errors are the number one cause of death and injury in the United States... ... over 784,000 people die annually due to medical mistakes. Comparatively, the 2001 annual death rate for heart disease was 699,697 and the annual death rate for cancer was 553,251.
>
> Over 2.2 million people are injured every year by prescription drugs alone and over 20 million unnecessary prescriptions for antibiotics are prescribed annually for viral infections. The report also shows that 7.5 million unnecessary medical and surgical procedures are performed every year and 8.9 million people are needlessly hospitalized annually. Based on the results of NIA's report, it is evident that there is a pressing need for an overhaul of the entire American medical system.

Even if one considers this particular report biased, it still reveals a trend in modern medicine: abuse of power by health professionals, abuse of trust, abuse of funds, abuse of patients' health, cost and treatment inefficiency. The more expensive med care gets, the more ineffective it seems to become. It is obvious: the health care system is failing, it is failing us, it is failing the purposes it was created for.

But why?

Because of the parasites and the predators. Health care has

become an industry. It is manufacturing thousands of medical professionals through a dehumanized educational system; it is producing trillions of "collateral profits" for the Big Pharma. The health care system has become vulnerable and weak against outside influences and machinations. It is not working anymore because it simply does not serve the purposes it was created to fulfill; it is not covering the needs it was designed to meet. It has become a health-broker, an envoy of the pharmaceutical world. It is not serving anyone else except itself and Big Pharma. And in its inner weakness it has become voracious. It is dictating, attacking, imposing. The average man is unprotected and lost in a labyrinth of mutual benefits and interests, arrangements and settlements that exclude him, in a system that was meant to protect and guide and keep him healthy. Public health is just an alibi for ever bigger business and despite its reclamations and affirmations, it is not public at all. It is very, very private, owned and defined by few.

Health is not a product. It is every man's birthright.

Is anybody, legislator, businessman or expert, entitled to defining and owning your very own health? The health of your family, the health of your fellow man? Should anyone be allowed to play mind games and gamble recklessly with your health?

Mass vaccinations, mass production of drugs, mass directives, mass profits. It is all about mass, muscles and volume. The people have become the phytoplankton for the gluttonous med care system. They abound, and even if overexploited they will find a way to replenish themselves.

This notion of mass health, of mass production of drugs is catastrophic. It may serve the industry; it does not serve the people. The invention of the median man, this populist, communist approach to public health is catastrophic. We are all different – to be treated with the same fashion as persons or as patients is simply ridiculous. Drugs that are good for you may kill me, drugs that are good for a mother may destroy her son. We are running out of patience and good intentions towards that oversimplifying mass medicine that is completely disregarding the individuality and the uniqueness of the person and of the organism.

In the meantime, populist medicine turns to popular drugs and popular diseases for profit. This Pulp Medicine neglects and ignores everything that doesn't have the potential to become an instant hit on the medical billboard. That is, Pulp Medicine looks down on rare health conditions. There is no glory and no profit in them. People with rare health conditions are usually excluded from med care planning, medical research and from drug development.

That was exactly the condition the Odones had to face. Indifference and disregard. Augusto and Michaela had a son, Lorenzo. And their son had a disease, not a disease like ODD and ADHD. A very real, very rare and terrible disease: ADL, Adrenoleukodystrophy, a neurodegenerating disease that can gradually can turn you into a vegetable.

Because the disease was rare, the Odones could find neither help nor comfort. For them, Pulp Med did not exist, or rather Pulp Med did not include them and their son. They were the "unfit".

Instead of giving up hope, blame fate or God and just despair and accept the "expert" death sentence their son received immediately after he was diagnosed with ADL, the Odones did the unthinkable: they took matters into their own hands and decided to succeed where everyone else had failed them.

Armed with Love, courage, dedication and reason they virtually moved into libraries, gathered every available data on their son's condition, brought together specialists, creating their own conference for their son's sake. The Odones turned the wheel and finally they were rewarded with an answer and a drug: an oil, Lorenzo's oil, that reduced fatty acid concentration on the brain, restricting thus the nerve cell demyelination that was resulting in ADL. They even talked a pharmaceutical company into producing the oil for their son and those in need of it. Unfortunately enough, tragic enough, it was kind of too late for Lorenzo: the oil could not reverse the brain damage that had already occurred. Despite that tragedy, the Odones managed to keep Lorenzo with them, to keep him alive and loved until the time of his death. Due to the tolls and the efforts of his loving parents, Lorenzo outlived the experts' death sentence he was given for 22 years. Thanks to him and his parents, other children with the same condition and their families enjoyed the preventive action of the oil and were probably spared a short life without a future, without hope, joy, expectations, achievements, dignity.

Even if Lorenzo suffered a cruel fate, the Odones can have their conscience at ease because they did everything that was humanly possible to save him, much, much more than what Pulp Med was willing and able to do for him and other children with his condition.

Were the Odones passionate? Off course they were. Did that passion hinder them from doing the best for their son? On the contrary, it kept them to their feet when everything around them was falling apart. The Odones are not only an example for patients and their families all over the world. They should be an example for medical practitioners and researchers all around the world. The goldfish science and the lab-rat science that disguise lack of inspiration and wit as impartiality and objectivity are at an end. Passion, when not interfering with the power of reasoning, is a desired human and scientific quality.

The Odones' example was followed by others. The Gelblooms had also a child and their child was also suffering from a rare neurodegenerating disease: Canavan Disease. Like the Odones, the Gelblooms rejected the rejection they received from Pulp Med and decided to dedicate themselves to finding answers and perhaps a cure. They gathered money, DNA samples, ignited research interest only to face an unjust patenting system that was denying them of the fruits of their labor.

It is obvious that the health care system has to be reformed. And whether this reform is to bear fruits or just create impressions to ease up the public opinion depends not only on the intensions and the vision of legislators and experts, but also on the active participation of the citizens. For too long, the average people, the median people, pleaded ignorance. We don't have time to get educated in medical issues; we don't have the data or the wit to make informed medical decisions. Damn, we don't even have the time to read the drug's side effects and indications. We are too medically illiterate to do anything like that. Let's leave it to the experts, at least they know what they are doing.

Greed and injustice thrives on apathy and indifference. Because the public got disinterested in science and medicine, the experts and the industries were left unchecked at a point where they had to account for nothing. Society's disregard towards science and medicine was repaid with science's disregard towards society and health.

We are all equal but still all wonderfully different. The new model of public health should be a personalized model at large. No longer should we tolerate being treated as uniform masses, or manipulated medical consumers. And the citizens should actively participate in research and science, become medically literate, responsibly informed, create groups and NGOs to promote their own interests, fund their own research and not only contribute in the vague symbolism and machine of the stock markets. The citizen should be once again be self-empowered, allowed to make his own decisions, of course under the guidance and advice of health experts. We are not abolishing health experts and health professionals. They are absolutely essential and sometimes an expert might be more knowledgeable than an entire society of people. The argument is that health authorities should not be allowed to become authoritarian.

The argument is that we should care for medicine if we anticipate science and medicine to care for us. It is a living relationship between science and society. Both parts have to tend for it and strive to preserve a working relationship.

The model of an active and well-educated citizen, of institutions that will respect and take into account the individuality, even in its biological aspect, of industries that will make profits from producing social and medical usefulness is the only working relationship. A relationship of mutual respect and mutual interest, a relationship of reciprocity. All else are cheap excuses and smokescreens created to hide dangerous personal ambitions and antisocial financial interests.

As David Healy profoundly described, we need a "new contract between society and the pharmaceutical industry – a contract that will require access to the raw data."

We are also in desperate need of a new contract between science, society, the individual and our culture.

# References

1    Rosenzweig P., Brohier S., Zipfel A., "The placebo effect in healthy volunteers: influence of the experimental conditions on the adverse events profile during phase I studies", Clin Pharmacol Ther 1993; 54:578-83.

2    Schweiger A., Parducci A., Pav J., "Nocebo: the psychologic induction of pain", Biol Sci 1981; 16:140-3.

3    Everson S.A., Kaplan G.A., Goldberg D.E., Salonen R., Jukka T., "Hopelessness and 4-year progression of carotid atherosclerosis: the Kuopio ischemic heart disease risk factor study", Arterioscler Thromb Biol 1997; 17:1490-5.

4    Glassman A.H., Shapiro A., "Depression and the course of coronary artery disease", Am J Psychiatry 1998; 155:4-11;
     Smith T.W., Ruiz J.M., "Psychosocial influences on the development and course of coronary heart disease: current status and implications for research and practice", J Consult Clin Psychol 2002 Jun; 73(3):459-62.

5    Pollitt R.A., Daniel M., Kaufman J.S., Lynch J.W., Salonen, J.T., Kaplan G.A., "Mediation and modification of the association between hopelessness, hostility and progression of carotid atherosclerosis", J Behav Med 2005 Feb; 28(1):53-64.

6    Schliefer S.J., Keller S.E., Camerino M.,Thornton J.C., Stein M., "Suppression of lymphocyte stimulation following bereavement", J Am Med Assoc (JAMA) 1983; 250:374-7.

7    "Past and present of 'what will please the lord': an updated history of the concept of placebo", Minerva Med 2005 Apr; 96(2):121-4.

8    Graves T.C., "Commentary on a Case of Hystero-Epilepsy with Delayed Puberty: Treated with Testicular Extract", The Lancet 1920 Dec 4; 196(5075).

9    Evans W. and Hoyle C., "The Comparative Value of Drugs Used in the Continuous Treatment of Angina Pectoris", Quarterly Journal of Medicine 1933 Jul; 2(7).

10   Gold H., Kwit N.T., Otto H., "The xanthines (theobromine and aminophylline) in the treatment of cardiac pain", JAMA 1937 Jun 26; 108(26):2173-79.

11   Jellinek E.M., "Clinical Tests on Comparative Effectiveness of Analgesic Drugs", Biometrics Bulletin 1946 Oct; 2(5):87-91.

12   Beecher H.K., "The powerful placebo", JAMA 1955 Dec 24; 159(17):1602-6.

13   Kirsch, Irving and Sapirstein, Guy, "Listening to Prozac but hearing placebo: A meta-analysis of antidepressant medication", Prevention & Treatment 1998 Jun; 1(1).

14   Hróbjartsson A., Gotzsche P.C., "Is the Placebo Powerless? An Analysis of Clinical Trials Comparing Placebo with No Treatment", New England J Med (NEJM) 2001 May 24; 344(21):1594-602.

15   Hróbjartsson A., Gotzsche P.C., "Is the placebo powerless? Update of a systematic review with 52 new randomized trials comparing placebo with no treatment", J Intern Med 2004 Aug; 256(2):91-100.

16   Blackwell B., Bloomfield S.S., Buncher C., "Demonstration to medical students of placebo responses and non-drug factors", The Lancet 1972; 13:1-11;
     Buckalew L.W., Coffield K.E., "An investigation of drug expectancy as a function of capsule colour and size and preparation form", J Clin Psychopharmacol 1982; 2:245-8.

17   Klopfer, Bruno, "Psychological variables in human cancer", Journal of Projective Techniques and Personality Assessment 1957; 21:331-34.

18   "Placebo Effect Can Last For Years", The New York Times, April 16, 1997

19   Benedetti F., Amanzio M., Baldi S., Casadio C., Cavallo A., Mancuso M., Ruffini E., Oliaro A., Maggi G., "The specific effects of prior opioid exposure on placebo analgesia and placebo respiratory depression", Pain 1998 Apr; 75(2-3):313-9.

20   "Placebo effect shocks allergy drugs maker", BBC News, July 5, 1999.

21   Talbot, Margaret, "The Placebo Prescription", The New York

Times, January 9, 2000.

22    Harrington, Anne (ed.), The Placebo Effect: An Interdisciplinary Exploration, Harvard University Press, Cambridge, 1997

23    Hahn R.A., "The Nocebo Phenomenon: The Concept, Evidence, and Implications for Public Health", Preventive Medicine 1997 Sep-Oct; 26(5):607-11;
Spiegel H., "Nocebo: The Power of Suggestibility", Preventive Medicine 1997 Sep-Oct; 26(5):616-21;
Barsky A.J. et al, "Nonspecific Medication Side Effects and the Nocebo Phenomenon", JAMA 2002 Feb; 287(5):622-27;

24    Fieschi D., "Criteri anatomo-fisiologici per intervento chirurgico lieve in malati di infarto e cuore di angina", Arch Ital Chir 1942; 63: 305-10.

25    Cobb L.A., Thomas G.I., Dillard D.H., Merendino K.A., Bruce R.A., "An evaluation of internal-mammary-artery ligation by a double-blind technique", NEJM 1959 May 28; 260(22):1115-18.

26    Moseley J.B., O'Malley K., Petersen N.J., Menke T.J., Brody B.A., Kuykendall D.H., Hollingsworth J.C., Ashton C.M., Wray N.P., "A controlled trial of arthroscopic surgery for osteoarthritis of the knee", NEJM 2002 Jul 11; 347(2):81-8.

27    Moseley J.B. Jr, Wray N.P., Kuykendall D., Willis K., Landon G., "Arthroscopic treatment of osteoarthritis of the knee: a prospective, randomized, placebo-controlled trial. Results of a pilot study", Am J Sports Med 1996 Jan-Feb; 24(1):28-34.

28    McRae C., Cherin E., Yamazaki T.G., Diem G., Vo A.H., Russell D., Ellgring J.H., Fahn S., Greene P., Dillon S., Winfield H., Bjugstad K.B., Freed C.R., "Effects of perceived treatment on quality of life and medical outcomes in a double-blind placebo surgery trial", Arch Gen Psychiatry 2004 Apr;61(4):412-20; Erratum in Arch Gen Psychiatry 2004 Jun; 61(6):627.

29    Benedetti F., "The opposite effects of the opiate antagonist naloxone and the cholecystokinin antagonist proglumide on placebo analgesia", Pain 1996 Mar;64(3):535-43.

30    Wager T.D., Rilling J.K., Smith E.E., Sokolik A., Casey K.L.,

Davidson R.J., Kosslyn S.M., Rose R.M., Cohen J.D., "Placebo induced changes in FMRI in the anticipation and experience of pain", Science 2004 Feb 20; 303(5661):1162-7;

Lieberman M.D., Jarcho J.M., Berman S., Naliboff B.D., Suyenobu B.Y., Mandelkern M., Mayer E.A., "The neural correlates of placebo effects: a disruption account", NeuroImage 2004 May; 22(1):447-55.

31   Pollo A., Vighetti S., Rainero I., Benedetti F., "Placebo analgesia and the heart", Pain 2003 Mar; 102(1-2):125-33;

Benedetti F., Amanzio M., Baldi S., Casadio C., Cavallo A., Mancuso M., Ruffini E., Oliaro A., Maggi G., "The specific effects of prior opioid exposure on placebo analgesia and placebo respiratory depression", Pain 1998 Apr; 75(2 3):313 9.

32   Gavin, Kara, "Thinking the pain away? U-M brain-scan study shows the body's own painkillers may cause the 'placebo effect'", University of Michigan press release, August 23, 2005.

33   Mayberg H.S., Silva J.A., Brannan S.K., Tekell J.L., Mahurin R.K., McGinnis S., Jerabek P.A., "The functional neuroanatomy of the placebo effect", Am J Psychiatry 2002 May; 159(5):728-37.

34   De la Fuente-Fernandez R., Phillips A.G., Zamburlini M., Sossi V., Calne D.B., Ruth T.J., Stoessl A.J., "Dopamine release in human ventral striatum and expectation of reward", Behav Brain Res 2002 Nov 15; 136(2):359-63.

35   Benedetti F., Colloca L., Torre E., Lanotte M., Melcarne A., Pesare M., Bergamasco B., Lopiano L., "Placebo-responsive Parkinson patients show decreased activity in single neurons of subthalamic nucleus", Nat Neurosci 2004 Jun; 7(6):587-8

36   Lynoe N., "Placebo is not always effective against nocebo bacilli. The body-mind interplay still wrapped in mystery", Läkartidningen 2005 Sep 19-25; 102(38):2627-8

37   Zajicek G., "The placebo effect is the healing force of nature", The Cancer Journal 1995 Mar-Apr; 8(2).

38   Wolf S., "Effects of Suggestion and Conditioning on the Action of Chemical Agents in Human Subjects: The Pharmacology of Placebos", Journal of Clinical Investigation, 1950 Jan; 29(1):100-109

39  ibid

40  http://www.aap.org/advocacy/releases/july08lipidscreening.htm

41  Rosuvastatin to Prevent Vascular Events in Men and Women with Elevated C-Reactive Protein, The Jupiter study group, NEJM 359:2195-2207, November 20, 2008

42  Ray Moynihan and Alan Cassels, Selling Sickness: How the World's Pharmaceutical Companies Are Turning Us All Into Patients, Nation Books, 2005

43  Leslie R. Wagstaff, Pharm.D., Melinda W. Mitton, Pharm.D., Beth McLendon Arvik, Pharm.D., P. Murali Doraiswamy, M.D. Statin-Associated Memory Loss: Analysis of 60 Case Reports and Review of the Literature Pharmacotherapy, July 25 2003.

44  Medical Tribune 15-30 June 2004, p 3

45  Vasankari T.J., Kujala U.M., Vasankari T.M., Ahotupa M. Reduced oxidized LDL levels after a 10-month exercise program. Med Sci Sports Exerc.(10):1496-501, 30 October 1998

46  Durstine J.L. & Haskell W.L. 1994. "Effects of exercise training on plasma lipids and lipoproteins". Exercise and Sports Science Reviews. 22:477-522.

47  Penny M. Kris-Etherton; William S. Harris; Lawrence J. Appel, Omega-3 Fatty Acids and Cardiovascular Disease, New Recommendations from the American Heart Association, Arteriosclerosis, Thrombosis, and Vascular Biology. 2003; 23:15

48  For a more detailed and competent chronicle of the Fen Phen destruction read Kate Cohen's Fen Phen Nation

49  http://www.who.int/medicines/areas/quality_safety/safety_effic acy/who_emp_qsm2008.3. pdf

50  http://news.bbc.co.uk/2/hi/health/4490271.stm Worldwide cancer cases 'double', Thursday, 28 April, 2005

51  http://www.who.int/mediacentre/news/releases/2003/pr27/en Global cancer could increase by 50% to a 15 million by 2020

52  http://www.un.org/esa/population/publications/worldageing 19502050

53  http://news.bbc.co.uk/2/hi/health/4079343.stm Child cancers

steadily increasing

54 http://www.who.int/mediacentre/news/releases/2003/pr27/en Global cancer could increase by 50% to a 15 million by 2020

55 Vessels of Death or Life By Rakesh K. Jain and Peter F. Carmeliet, Scientific American December 2001

56 http://www.who.int/mediacentre/news/releases/2003/pr27/en Global cancer could increase by 50% to a 15 million by 2020

57 http://www.newsweek.com/id/157548 We fought cancer... and cancer won, by Sharon Begley, September 6, 2008

58 http://money.cnn.com/magazines/fortune/fortune_archive/2004/03/22/365076/index.htm Why we are losing the war on cancer, by Clifton Leaf, March 22 2004

59 Ibid

60 http://www.newsweek.com/id/157548 We fought cancer... and cancer won, by Sharon Begley, September 6 2008

61 http://www.cnn.com/2007/HEALTH/01/09/fortune.leaf.waron-cancer3/index.html by Clifton Leaf

62 The BRCA1/2 pathway prevents hematologic cancers in addition to breast and ovarian cancers, Friedenson B., BMC Cancer 7: 152

63 http://news.bbc.co.uk/2/hi/health/8116790.stm New cancer drug shows promise, June 24 2009

64 Target Practice: Lessons from Phase III Trials with Bevacizumab and Vatalanib in the treatment of advanced colorectal cancer. Los M., Roodhart J.M., Voest E.E., The Oncologist 12 (4): 443–50

65 http://www.forbes.com/forbes/2009/0302/074_cancer_miracles.html Cancer Miracles, by Robert Langreth

66 http://www.medarex.com/cgi-local/item.pl/20071210-1085876

67 http://www.forbes.com/forbes/2009/0302/074_cancer_miracles.html Cancer Miracles, by Robert Langreth

68 http://health.eportal.gr/health/themataoz_ereynes/15698oz_2007090115698.php3

69 http://www.cancer.gov/cancertopics/types/prostate

70 http://news.bbc.co.uk/2/hi/health/5304910.stm Gene therapy rids man of cancer

71 Carnesecchi S., et al, 2001, Geraniol, a Component of Plant Essential Oils, Inhibits Growth and Polyamine Biosynthesis in Human Colon Cancer Cells, Pharmacology, Vol. 298, Issue 1, 197-200, July 2001

72 ibid

73 Elson and Yu, 1994, The chemoprevention of cancer by mevalonate-derived constituents of fruits and vegetables. J Nutr 124: 607-614; Kelloff, et al, 1996, Kelloff G.J., et al, 1996, New agents for cancer chemoprevention, J Cell Biochem 26: 1-28; Crowell, 1999, Crowell PL, 1999, Prevention and therapy of cancer by dietary monoterpenes, J Nutr 129: 775S-778S

74 Elegbede et al, 1986, Mouse skin tumor promoting activity of orange peel oil and d-limonene: a re-evaluation, Carcinogenesis 7: 2047-2049; Wattenberg and Coccia, 1991, Inhibition of 4-(methylnitrosamino)-1-(3-pyridyl)-1-butanone carcinogenesis in mice by D-limonene and citrus fruit oils, Carcinogenesis 12: 115-117; Crowell and Gould, 1994, Chemoprevention and therapy of cancer by d-limonene, Crit Rev Oncog, 5: 1-22 ; Mills et al, 1995, Induction of apoptosis in liver tumors by the monoterpene perillyl alcohol, Cancer Res 55: 979-983; Kawamori et al, 1996, Inhibitory effects of d-limonene on the development of colonic aberrant crypt foci induced by azoxymethane in F344 rats, Carcinogenesis, 17: 369-372

75 Haag and Gould, 1994, Mammary carcinoma regression induced by perillyl alcohol, a hydroxylated analog of limonene, Cancer Chemother Pharmacol, 34: 477-483; Stark et al, 1995, Chemotherapy of pancreatic cancer with the monoterpene perillyl alcohol, Cancer Lett, 96: 15-21; Reddy et al, 1997, Chemoprevention of colon carcinogenesis by dietary perillyl alcohol, Cancer Res, 57: 420-425

76 Shoff et al, 1991, Concentration-dependent increase of murine P388 and B16 population doubling time by the acyclic monoterpene geraniol, Cancer Res, 51: 37-42; Yu et al, 1995, Geraniol, an inhibitor of mevalonate biosynthesis, suppresses the

growth of hepatomas and melanomas transplanted to rats and mice, J Nutr, 125: 2763-2767; Burke et al, 1997, Inhibition of pancreatic cancer growth by the dietary isoprenoids farnesol and geraniol, Lipids, 32: 151-156: ref Carnesecchi S et al, 2001, Geraniol, a Component of Plant Essential Oils, Inhibits Growth and Polyamine Biosynthesis in Human Colon Cancer Cells, Pharmacology, Vol. 298, Issue 1, 197-200, July 200

77   Dean A., et al, 2006, Cell Cycle Arrest by the Isoprenoids Perillyl Alcohol, Geraniol, and Farnesol Is Mediated by p21$^{Cip1}$ and p27$^{Kip1}$ in Human Pancreatic Adenocarcinoma Cells, Journal of Pharmacology And Experimental Therapeutics Fast Forward, First published on November 30, 2006; DOI: 10.1124/jpet.106.111666

78   Lynn Sagan "On the origin of mitosing cells". J Theor Bio. 14 (3): 255–274 (1967)

79   http://www.ninds.nih.gov/news_and_events/proceedings/2009 0629_mitochondrial.htm

80   B.B. Burnett, A. Gardner, R.G. Boles. "Mitochondrial inheritance in depression, dysmotility and migraine?" J Affect Disord (2005) 88: 109-16

81   Gimsa U., Kanitz E., Otten W., Ibrahim S.M. "Behavior and stress reactivity in mouse strains with mitochondrial DNA variations." Ann N Y Acad Sci. 2009 Feb; 1153:131-8.

82   http://nass.oxfordjournals.org/cgi/reprint/2/1/253.pdf

83   Gardner A. and Boles R.G., "Mitochondrial Energy Depletion in Depression with Somatization" Psychotherapy and Psychosomatics 77:127-129

84   http://www.blackwellpublishing.com/eccmid16/abstract.asp?id= 49195

85   http://www8.utsouthwestern.edu/utsw/cda/dept37389/files/2379 73.html

86   John A. Lewis, Afroza Huq and Pilar Najarro, "Inhibition of Mitochondrial Function by Interferon", the Journal of Biological Chemistry, May 31, 1996 271, 13184-13190

87   "Anti-mitochondrial type M5 and anti-cardiolipin antibodies in

autoimmune disorders: studies on their association and cross-reactivity." P.L. Meroni, E.N. Harris, A. Brucato, A. Tincani, W. Barcellini, A. Vismara, G. Balestrieri, G.R. Hughes, and C. Zanussi, Clin Exp Immunol. 1987 March; 67(3): 484–491.
"Anti-phospholipid and anti-mitochondrial type M5 antibodies in systemic lupus erythematosus." Tincani A., Meroni P..L, Brucato A., Zanussi C., Allegri F., Mantelli P., Cattaneo R., Balestrieri G., Clin Exp Rheumatol. 1985 Oct–Dec; 3(4):321–326

88   J. Bereiter-Hahn, Intracellular motility of mitochondria: role of the inner compartment in migration and shape changes of mitochondria in XTH-cell Journal of Cell Science, Vol 30, Issue 1 99-115

89   http://www.mitochondrial.net/showabstract.php?pmid=19745815, an exciting site devoted to mitochondrial research and news

90   Changes in the human mitochondrial genome after treatment of malignant disease. T.M. Wardell, E. Ferguson, P.F. Chinnery, G.M. Borthwick, R.W. Taylor, G. Jackson, A. Craft, R.N. Lightowlers, N. Howell, D.M. Turnbull, Mutat Res (2003) 525: 19-27.

91   Mitochondrial damage in muscle occurs after marked depletion of glutathione and is prevented by giving glutathione monoester. Mårtensson J., Meister A., Proc Nat'l Acad Sci U S A. 1989 Jan; 86(2):471-5

92   http://www.blackwellpublishing.com/eccmid19/abstract.asp?id =74880

93   "Mitochondrial toxic effects and ribavirin" Dominique Salmon-Céron, Laurence Chauvelot-Moachon, Sébastien Abad, Benjamin Silbermann, Philippe Sogni, The Lancet, Volume 357, Issue 9270, 1803 - 1804, 2 June 2001

94   http://www.psmid.org.ph/vol15/vol15num2topic9.pdf

95   http://aac.asm.org/cgi/reprint/51/1/54.pdf

96   http://www.ninds.nih.gov/news_and_events/proceedings/20090 629_mitochondrial.htm

97   Food supplements found to reverse the ageing process, By Steve Connor, The Independent, Tuesday, 19 February 2002

98   "Thiamine for the treatment of nucleoside analogue-induced severe lactic acidosis" C. Schramm, R. Wanitschke and P.R. Galle, European Journal of Anaesthesiology (1999), 16:10:733-735

99   How Yeast Can Create Havoc in Your Life and How to Address it, Dr. Mercola, December 2, 2008

100  M.L.F. van Velthuysen and S. Florquin, Jan 2000, Clin Microbiol Rev. 13(1): 55–66

101  Aranka Anema and Koert Ritmeijer, Synopsis, Treating Leishmaniasis and HIV/AIDS Co-infection in Ethiopia, May 24, 2005, CMAJ 172 (11)

102  Alvar J., Gutierrez-Solar B., Molina R., Lopez-Velez R., Garcia-Camacho A., Martinez P. et al. Prevalence of Leishmania infection among AIDS patients [letter]. Lancet 1992; 339: 1427

103  Aranka Anema and Koert Ritmeijer, Synopsis, Treating Leishmaniasis and HIV/AIDS Co-infection in Ethiopia, May 24, 2005, CMAJ 172 (11)

104  S. Sundar, N.K. Aggarwal, P.R. Sihna, G.S. Horwith, H.W. Murray, July 1997, Short-Course, Low-Dose Amphotericin B Lipid Complex Therapy for Visceral Leishmaniasis Unresponsive to Antimony, Annals of Internal Medicine, Vol 127 (20, 133-137

105  H.W. Murray, August 2001, Clinical and Experimental Advances in Treatment of Visceral Leishmaniasis, AMS, Vol 5 No 8, 2185-2197

106  Florence T.M., Centre for Environmental and Health Science Pty Ltd, Sydney, NSW, Aust N Z J Ophthalmol 1995; 23(1) Feb: 3–7

107  Jean et al, Nutrition During and After Cancer Treatment: A Guide for Informed Choices by Cancer Survivors, CA Cancer J Clin 2001; 51:153-181© 2001 American Cancer Society

108  The Washington Post, Tuesday, February 15, 2005; Page HE01, Jim Morris

109  Chemicals Health Monitor, 5th June, 2009

110  ibid

111  Chemicals Health Monitor, 22nd June, 2009

112  Chemicals Health Monitor, 13th May, 2009

113  Yumiko et al, Human Reproduction, Determination of bisphenol A

concentrations in human biological fluids reveals significant early prenatal exposure, Human Reproduction, Vol. 17, No. 11, 2839-2841, November 2002

114 Rider et al, Cumulative Effects of In Utero Administration of Mixtures of "Antiandrogens" on Male Rat Reproductive Development, Toxicol Path, 2009;37(1):100-13

115 Gray et al, Administration of potentially antiandrogenic pesticides (procymidone, linuron, iprodione, chlozolinate, p,p'-DDE, and ketoconazole) and toxic substances (dibutyl- and diethylhexyl phthalate, PCB 169, and ethane dimethane sulphonate) during sexual differentiation produces diverse profiles of reproductive malformations in the male rat, Toxicol Ind Health, 1999 Jan-Mar;15(1-2):94-118

116 Bello et al, Characterization of occupational exposures to cleaning products used for common cleaning tasks – a pilot study of hospital cleaners, Environ Health, 2009 Mar 27;8:11.

117 Zhang et al, Formaldehyde exposure and leukemia: a new meta-analysis and potential mechanisms, Mutat Res, 2009 Mar-Jun; 681(2-3):150-68, Epub 2008 Jul 15

118 http://www.newmediaexplorer.org/sepp/

119 ibid

120 Goran Bjelakovic et al, Mortality in Randomized Trials of Antioxidant Supplements for Primary and Secondary Prevention Systematic Review and Meta-analysis, JAMA, February 28, 2007 — Vol 297, No. 8 847-857

121 ibid

122 Hercberg et al, The potential role of antioxidant vitamins in preventing cardiovascular diseases and cancers, Nutrition. 1998; 14:513-520

123 Goran Bjelakovic et al, Mortality in Randomized Trials of Antioxidant Supplements for Primary and Secondary Prevention Systematic Review and Meta-analysis, JAMA, February 28, 2007 — Vol 297, No. 8 847-857

124 Leaf A., Circulation. 2003; 107:2646, 2003 American Heart

237

Association, Inc

125   Ann Intern Med. 2005 Jan 4; 142(1):37-46

126   Heinonen OP et al, The effect of vitamin E and beta-carotene on the incidence of lung cancer and other cancers in male smokers, New England J of Med 330:1029-1035, 1994

127   Boundary violation and sexual exploitation in psychiatry and psychotherapy: a review
      Sameer P. Sarkar Advances in Psychiatric Treatment (2004) 10: 312-320

128   Against therapy, by Jeffrey Masson, Atheneum 1988.

129   The Interpretation of Dreams, Sigmund Freud, Avon Books

130   New Introductory Lectures on Psycho-analysis, Sigmund Freud

131   Conjectures and Refutations, Karl Popper, London: Routledge and Keagan Paul, 1963

132   The Hitchhiker's Guide to the Galaxy, Douglas Adams, Ballantine Books, 1995


133   http://www.time.com/time/magazine/article/0,9171,1074806-1,00.html, Battling over Masochism, by John Leo

134   Beyond Freedom and Dignity, B.F. Skinner, Cape, 1975

135   http://www.moshersoteria.com/resig.htm Letter of resignation from the American Psychiatric Association, Loren R. Mosher

136   Epidemiology of Affective Disorders: A Review, Bland, R.C., Can J Psychiatry 42: 367?377

137   Alternative projections of mortality and disability by cause 1990-2020: Global Burden of Disease study, Murray C.J., Lopez A.D., Lancet 1997, vol. 349, n°9064, pp. 1498-1504

138   Depression, suicide, and the national service framework, Davies S., Naik P.C., Lee A.S., BMJ 2001; 322: 1501-2

139   http://www.moshersoteria.com/resig.htm Letter of resignation from the American Psychiatric Association, Loren R. Mosher

140   Kirsch, Irving; Sapirstein, Guy. Listening to Prozac but hearing placebo: A meta-analysis of antidepressant medication, Prevention & Treatment. 1(1), Jun 1998

141  Initial Severity and Antidepressant Benefits: A Meta-Analysis of Data Submitted to the Food and Drug Administration, Irving Kirsch et al, PLoS Medicine 5(2): e45

142  http://money.cnn.com/magazines/fortune/fortune_archive/2005 /11/28/8361973/index.htm Trouble in Prozac, by David Stipp

143  Serotonin and Depression: A Disconnect between the Advertisements and the Scientific Literature. Lacasse J.R., Leo J., PLoS Med 2(12): e392

144  http://www.news-medical.net/news/2005/11/13/14435.aspx Adverts for SSRI antidepressants misleading

145  Serotonin and Depression: A Disconnect between the Advertisements and the Scientific Literature. Lacasse J.R., Leo J., PLoS Med 2(12): e392

146  ibid

147  http://money.cnn.com/magazines/fortune/fortune_archive/2005 /11/28/8361973/index.htm Trouble in Prozac, by David Stipp

148  http://www.publications.parliament.uk/pa/cm200405/cmselect /cmhealth/42/4202.htm United Kingdom Parliament (2005) House of Commons health report. London: United Kingdom House of Commons

149  Exercise treatment for depression: efficacy and dose response. Dunn A.L., Trivedi M.H., Kampert J.B., Clark C.G., Chambliss H.O., Am J Prev Med. 2005 Jan; 28(1):1-8.

150  http://www.dukenews.duke.edu/2000/09/exercise922.html Study: Exercise Has Long-Lasting Effect on Depression, September 22, 2000

151  http://www.moshersoteria.com/resig.htm Letter of resignation from the American Psychiatric Association, Loren R. Mosher

152  ibid

153  And They Call It Help: The Psychiatric Policing of America's Children, Louise Armstrong, Addison-Wesley, 1993

154  Political Apathy Disorder: Proposal for a New DSM Diagnostic Category, Geoffrey D.White, Journal of Humanistic Psychology.2004; 44: 47-57

155 http://www.huffingtonpost.com/dennis-palumbo/do-you-suffer-from-politi_b_160162.html

156 Scientists find new disease: motivational deficiency disorder, Ray Moynihan, BMJ.2006; 332: 745

157 Making Us Crazy: DSM, the Psychiatric Bible and the Creation of Mental Disorders. – book reviews, by E. Fuller Torrey, M.D., Washington Monthly, Jan-Feb 1998

158 Bedlam: Greed, Profiteering, and Fraud in a Mental Health System Gone Crazy, Joe Sharkey, St. Martin's Press, 1994

159 http://www.newsweek.com/id/108730 Baseball's other drug problem, by Charles Euchner, February 6, 2008

160 ibid

161 Companion to Clinical Neurology. William Pryse-Phillips, Oxford University Press 2003

162 http://www.moshersoteria.com/resig.htm Letter of resignation from the American Psychiatric Association, Loren R. Mosher

163 http://www.scribd.com/doc/13463979/Fear-and-Loathing-in-Cannabis-Country

164 Cannabis-induced psychosis and subsequent schizophrenia-spectrum disorders: follow-up study of 535 incident cases, Mikkel Arendt, MScPsych; Raben Rosenberg, DMSci; Leslie Foldager, MSc; Gurli Perto, The British Journal of Psychiatry (2005) 187: 510-515

165 Suppression of the humoral immune response by cannabinoids is partially mediated through inhibition of adenylate cyclase by pertussis toxin-sensitive G-protein coupled mechanism Kaminski N.E., Koh W.S., Yang K.H., Lee M., Kessler F.K. Biochemical Pharmacology 1994, vol. 48, n°10, pp. 1899-1908

166 Cannabis-induced psychosis and subsequent schizophrenia-spectrum disorders: follow-up study of 535 incident cases Mikkel Arendt, MScPsych, Raben Rosenberg, DMSci, Leslie Foldager, MSc, Gurli Perto The British Journal of Psychiatry (2005) 187: 510-515

167 Direct suppression of CNS autoimmune inflammation via the cannabinoid receptor $CB_1$ on neurons and $CB_2$ on autoreactive T cells, Katarzyna Maresz, Gareth Pryce, Eugene D Ponomarev,

Giovanni Marsicano, J. Ludovic Croxford, Leah P Shriver, Catherine Ledent, Xiaodong Cheng, Erica J Carrier, Monica K. Mann, Gavin Giovannoni, Roger G. Pertwee, Takashi Yamamura, Nancy E. Buckley, Cecilia J. Hillard, Beat Lutz, David Baker & Bonnie N. Dittel, Nature Medicine 13, 492 - 497 (2007)

168 http://www.newscientist.com/article/dn12016-cannabis-compound-reduces-skin-allergies-in-mice.html

169 A Molecular Link Between the Active Component of Marijuana and Alzheimer's Disease Pathology. Eubanks L.M., Rogers C.J., Beuscher A.E. et al. (Nov 2006) Molecular Pharmaceutics 3 (6): 773–7.

170 Cannabinoids promote embryonic and adult hippocampus neurogenesis and produce anxiolytic- and antidepressant-like effects Jiang W., Zhang Y., Xiao L., et al, The Journal of Clinical Investigation 115 (11):3104–16 (November 2005)

171 American Association for Cancer Research (2007, April 17). Marijuana Cuts Lung Cancer Tumor Growth In Half, Study Shows

172 "Cannabidiol as a novel inhibitor of Id-1 gene expression in aggressive breast cancer cells", McAllister S.D., Christian R.T., Horowitz M.P., Garcia A., Desprez P.Y., Molecular Cancer Therapeutics 6 (11): 2921–7 (November 2007)

173 "Cannabinoid action induces autophagy-mediated cell death through stimulation of ER stress in human glioma cells", Salazar M., Carracedo A., Salanueva I.J., et al., the Journal of Clinical Investigation 119 (5): 1359–72 (May 2009).

174 "Dronabinol and marijuana in HIV-positive marijuana smokers. Caloric intake, mood, and sleep". Haney M., Gunderson E.W., Rabkin J., et al, Journal of Acquired Immune Deficiency Syndromes 45 (5): 545–54 (August 2007)

175 "Short-term effects of cannabinoids in patients with HIV-1 infection: a randomized, placebo-controlled clinical trial". Abrams D.I., Hilton J.F., Leiser R.J. et al. Annals of Internal Medicine 139 (4): 258–66. (August 2003)

176 New Review J. For. Sci. 46: 1138, 2001

177 J. For. Sci. 45: 843, 2000

178 Miller and Giannini, 1990, The disease model of addiction: a biopsychiatrist's view, J Psychoactive Drugs 22 (1): 83–5

179 Koob and Kreek, 2007, Stress, Dysregulation of Drug Reward Pathways, and the Transition to Drug Dependence, Am J Psychiatry 164 (8): 1149–59

180 Jones and Bonci, 2005, Synaptic plasticity and drug addiction, Curr Opin Pharmacol 5 (1): 20–5

181 Johnson R.E. et al, 2000, "A comparison of levomethadyl acetate, buprenorphine, and methadone for opioid dependence", N. Engl. J. Med. 343 (18): 1290–7: Connock M. et al, 2007, "Methadone and buprenorphine for the management of opioid dependence: a systematic review and economic evaluation", Health Technology Assessment 11 (9): 1–171, iii–iv

182 Kenna G.A. et al, 2007, Pharmacotherapy of dual substance abuse and dependence, CNS Drugs 21 (3): 213–37

183 International Journal of Pharmacology, 1975

184 http://www.healthreform.gov/reports/inaction/inactionreport-printmarch2009.pdf The costs of inaction, the urgent need for health reform

185 http://www.webdc.com/pdfs/deathbymedicine.pdf Death by medicine, 2004, Null G., Dean C, Feldman M., Rasio D., and Smith D.

186 Saunders PT. The depression side of medical science. Science in Society 39, 50-51, 2008

187 Saunders PT. Why the planet is sick. Science in Society 39, 50-51, 2008.

188 http://www.americanchiropractic.net/healthcare_general/Death%20of%20Medicine.pdf The death of medicine. No cure, no vaccine, no treatment. Regush N. 2002

189 http://www.i-sis.org.uk/unravelingAIDS.php Ho M.W., Burcher S., Gala R. and Voljkovic V. Unraveling AIDS, Vital Health Publishing, Ridgefield, CT, 2005.

190 Ho M.W. GM is Dangerous and Futile. Science in Society 40, 4-8,

2008

191  Ho M.W. Drowning in a Sea of Microwaves, the Wi-Fi Revolution. Science in Society 34, 11-13, 2007.

192  Burcher S. Picking Cotton Carefully. Science in Society 34, 21-23, 2007.

193  Ho M.W. Science in a New Key. Science in Society 43

194  Ho M.W., Burcher S., Lim L.C. et al. Food Futures Now, Organic, Sustainable, Fossil Fuel Free, ISIS/TWN, London/Penang, 2008, http://www.i-sis.org.uk/foodFutures.php

195  Ho M.W. From Genomics to Epigenomics. Science in Society 41, 10-12, 2009.

196  Schrödinger E. What is Life? Cambridge University Press, Cambridge 1944.

197  Ho M.W. The Rainbow and the Worm, the Physics of Organisms, World Scientific, Singapore, 1993, 2$^{nd}$ ed. 1998, reprinted 1999, 20021, 2003, 2005, 2006; 3$^{rd}$ ed. 2008. http://www.i-sis.org.uk/rnbwwrm.php

198  Watton A, Haffegee H, Burcher S and Ho MW. Quantum Jazz, a Fusion of contemporary jazz music and digital video recordings of live organisms, http://www.i-sis.org.uk/onlinestore/av.php

199  Ho M.W. Drowning in a Sea of Microwaves, the Wi-Fi revolution. Science in Society 34, 11-13, 2007.

200  Ho M.W. Quantum Jazz, the Tao of Biology. Science in Society 34, 17-20, 2007

201  Ho M.W. The Heartbeat of Health. Science in Society 35, 10-13, 2007.

202  Ho M.W. Happiness is a Heartbeat away. Science in Society 35, 14-18, 2007.

203  Ho M.W. Water Electric. Science in Society 43

204  Ho MW. Positive Electricity Zaps through Water Chains. Science in Society 28, 49-50, 2005.

205  Ho MW. Happiness is a Heartbeat away. Science in Society 35, 14-18, 2007.

206  Ho MW. The Real Bioinformatics Revolution. Proteins and Nucleic

Acids Singing to One Another? Science in Society 33, 42-45, 2007.

207 Oschman JL. Energy Medicine, The Scientific Basis, Churchill Livingston, New York, 2000.

208 Ho MW. Collagen Water Structure Revealed. Science in Society 32, 15-18, 2006.

209 Ho MW and Knight D. Liquid crystalline meridians. The American Journal of Chinese Medicine 1998, 26, 251-63. http://www.i-sis.org.uk/onlinestore/papers1.php#section3

210 Ho MW. Acupuncture, coherent energy and the liquid crystalline organism, Plenary Lecture, Second International Congress on Acupuncture, 2-5, June 2005, Barcelona, Spain, http://www.i-sis.org.uk/onlinestore/papers1.php#section4

211 Ho MW. Water Electric. Science in Society 43

212 Ho MW. Water and Fire series. Science in Society 43

213 Szent-Györgyi A. Oxidation, energy transfer, and vitamins, Nobel Lecture, 11 December 1937.

214 Cummins J. 'Biologicals' Wonder Drugs with Problems. Science in Society 42, 34-35, 2009.

215 Ho MW. Living with the Fluid Genome, ISIS TWN, London, 2003.

216 Ho MW. From Genomics to Epigenomics. Science in Society 41, 10-12, 2009.

217 Ho MW. Caring Mothers Strike Fatal Blow against Genetic Determinism. Science in Society 41, 6-9, 2009.

218 Switzerland enshrines complementary medicine in the constitution", 19 May 2009, Cybermed.It, http://www.cybermed.it/index2.php?option=com_content&do_pdf=1&id=22360

219 Oschman JL. Energy Medicine, The Scientific Basis, Churchill Livingston, New York, 2000.

# Bibliography

Marcia Angell – The Truth about the Drug Companies: How They Deceive Us and What to Do about It, Random House, 2004

Sigmund Freud
– The Interpretation of Dreams, Wordsworth Editions Ltd, 2000
– Introduction to Psychoanalysis

David Healy – Let Them Eat Prozac: The Unhealthy Relationship Between the Pharmaceutical Industry and Depression, NYU Press, 2004

Hermann Hesse – Steppenwolf, (latest hardcover edition: Amereon ltd, 1983)

Mae-Wan Ho
– Living with the Fluid Genome, Institute of Science in Society, 2003
– The Rainbow and the Worm, the Physics of Organisms, World Scientific, Singapore, 1993
– Turning the Tide on the Brave New World of Bad Science and Big Business, Continuum, 2000

Ivan Illich – Medical Nemesis – The Expropriation of Health, Marion Boyers, 1974

Thomas S. Kuhn – The Structure of Scientific Revolutions, University of Chicago Press, 1996

Ray Moynihan and Alan Cassels – Selling Sickness: How the World's Biggest Pharmaceutical Companies Are Turning Us All Into Patients, Nation Books, 2005

Oschman JL – Energy Medicine, The Scientific Basis, Churchill Livingston, New York, 2000

Lynn Payer – Disease-Mongers: How Doctors, Drug Companies and Insurers Are Making You Feel Sick by, John Wiley and Sons inc, 1994

Karl Popper – Conjectures and Refutations, , London: Routledge and Keagan Paul, 1963

Sheldon Rampton, John Stauber – Trust Us We're Experts: How Industry Manipulates Science and Gambles with Your Future, Penguin Putnam

Matthias Rath – Eradicating Heart Disease, Health Now, 1993

Janine Roberts – Fear of the invisible, Impact Investigative Media Productions, 2008

Joe Sharkey – Bedlam: Greed, Profiteering, and Fraud in a Mental Health System Gone Crazy, St. Martin's Press, 1994

B.F. Skinner – Beyond Freedom and Dignity, Cape, 1975

Thomas Szasz

– The Myth of Mental Illness: Foundations of a Theory of Personal Conduct. Harper & Row, 1974

– My Madness Saved Me: The Madness and Marriage of Virginia Woolf. Somerset NJ: Transaction Publishers, 2006

George Vithoulkas

– A New Model of Health and Disease, The International Academy of Classical Homeopathy

– Homeopathy- Medicine for the new millennium, The International Academy of Classical Homeopathy

Aaron Wildavsky – Searching for Safety, Social Philosophy and Policy Center, 1988

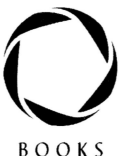

# BOOKS

O is a symbol of the world, of oneness and unity. In different cultures it also means the "eye," symbolizing knowledge and insight. We aim to publish books that are accessible, constructive and that challenge accepted opinion, both that of academia and the "moral majority."

Our books are available in all good English language bookstores worldwide. If you don't see the book on the shelves ask the bookstore to order it for you, quoting the ISBN number and title. Alternatively you can order online (all major online retail sites carry our titles) or contact the distributor in the relevant country, listed on the copyright page.

See our website **www.o-books.net** for a full list of over 500 titles, growing by 100 a year.

And tune in to myspiritradio.com for our book review radio show, hosted by June-Elleni Laine, where you can listen to the authors discussing their books.

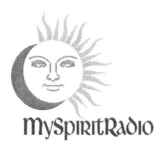

MySpiritRadio